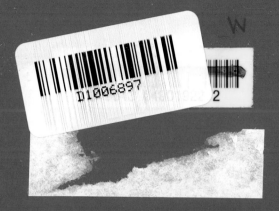

W

Strong Women, Strong Bones

◆ ◆ ◆

EVERYTHING YOU NEED
TO KNOW TO PREVENT,
TREAT, AND BEAT
OSTEOPOROSIS

G. P. Putnam's Sons
New York

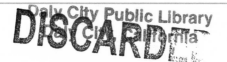
Strong Women, Strong Bones

◆ ◆ ◆

EVERYTHING YOU NEED
TO KNOW TO PREVENT,
TREAT, AND BEAT
OSTEOPOROSIS

◆ ◆ ◆

MIRIAM E. NELSON, PH.D.
with
SARAH WERNICK, PH.D.

W

616.716

NEL

G. P. Putnam's Sons
Publishers Since 1838
a member of
Penguin Putnam Inc.
375 Hudson Street
New York, NY 10014

Photo on page 18 copyright David W. Dempster, 1999.

Photos on page 33 reprinted with permission E. F. Eriksen, D. W. Axelrod, F. Melsen, *Bone Histomorphometry,* Raven Press, Ltd., 1994, pages 26–28.

Illustration on page 38 redrawn with permission from a photograph on page 230 of *The Wellness Guide to Lifelong Fitness* (Rebus, New York), by Timothy P. White, Ph.D., and the editors of the University of California at Berkeley *Wellness Letter.*

Photos on page 70 reprinted courtesy of Hologic, Inc.

Map on page 118 reprinted with permission *Tufts University Health & Nutrition Letter.*

PAR-Q questionnaire on pages 138 and 139, reprinted with permission Canadian Society for Exercise Physiology.

Every effort has been made to ensure that the information contained in this book is complete and accurate. However, neither the publisher nor the author is engaged in rendering professional advice or services to the individual reader. The ideas, procedures, and suggestions contained in this book are not intended as a substitute for consulting with your physician and obtaining medical supervision as to any activity, procedure, or suggestion that might affect your health. Accordingly, individual readers must assume responsibility for their own actions, safety, and health, and neither the author nor the publisher shall be liable or responsible for any loss, injury, or damage allegedly arising from any information or suggestion in this book.

Library of Congress Cataloging-in-Publication Data
Nelson, Miriam E.
Strong women, strong bones : everything you need to know to prevent, treat, and beat
osteoporosis / Miriam E. Nelson with Sarah Wernick; illustrations by Wendy Wray.
p.   cm.
Includes bibliographical references and index.
ISBN 0-399-14597-4
1. Osteoporosis in women—Popular works.   I. Wernick, Sarah.   II. Title.
RC931.O73 N45   2000   99-057570
616.7'16—dc21

Printed in the United States of America
1   3   5   7   9   10   8   6   4   2

This book is printed on acid-free paper. ∞

Book design by Deborah Kerner

FOR ALEXANDRA,
ELIZA,
AND MASON

An Important Caution

◆ ◆ ◆

The *Strong Women, Strong Bones* program is based on extensive scientific research. The book contains detailed instructions and safety precautions. It is essential that you read them carefully. Some exercises are inappropriate for individuals with bone loss or other medical problems.

This book is *not* intended to replace the services of a health-care provider who knows you personally. An essential element of taking responsibility for your health is having regular checkups and working in partnership with medical professionals.

If you are under treatment for osteoporosis or any other medical condition—or if you suspect you might need such care—you must discuss this program with a physician before you start.

Contents

◆ ◆ ◆

Acknowledgments

◆ ◆ ◆

This book would not have been possible without the help and expertise of many people. I want to express my thanks, respect, and gratitude to them.

My deep appreciation to Drs. Ronenn Roubenoff and Irwin Rosenberg. Their never-ending support for my work, and their belief in the importance of disseminating research, have made this book possible.

I am enormously grateful to the National Osteoporosis Foundation's Department of Patient and Professional Education for their careful review of the manuscript and their many helpful comments. Dr. Robert Neer read the entire book and thoughtfully provided numerous valuable clarifications and corrections. Drs. Joan Bassey, Sarah Booth, Bess Dawson-Hughes, Wendy Kohrt, Christine Snow, and Katherine Tucker gave me guidance on exercise, nutrition, and bone health through their important research. Drs. Kristin Baker, Melissa Bernstein, Christina Economos, and Carmen Castaneda Sceppa have always been at the ready for my questions about exercise and nutrition. Drs. Elizabeth Ross and Meryl LeBoff answered my inquiries on medication management.

I am especially indebted to Jennifer Layne, M.S., C.S.C.S. Jennifer's expertise is extraordinary. She made significant contributions to all three of my books, translating scientific research into effective, practical exercises.

Joseph Walsmith, M.S., was helpful in answering my questions on balance and falls. Rebecca Seguin and Karyn Roach provided invaluable assistance by gathering the research and developing various sections of the book.

I am so grateful to my publishing colleagues, who played a vital role in making this book possible. Sarah Wernick, my phenomenal collaborator and cherished friend, worked with great intelligence and diligence. Wendy Weil, my agent, has been a constant support throughout my writing endeavors. Wendy Wray, whose illustrations greatly enhanced my first two books, brought her keen eye and clear definition to the figures. I've been inspired by the enthusiastic support of Stacy Creamer, my energetic editor at Putnam, who successfully completed the Empire State Building Stair Challenge last year. It's been a pleasure working with her. I feel very fortunate to have had the thoughtful editorial input of three outstanding writers—Anita Bartholomew, Sally Wendkos Olds, and Barbara Sofer. Special thanks to my Tufts colleague Dr. William Lockeretz, who combed the entire manuscript with his usual care and perception.

My thanks to Larry Lindner and the *Tufts University Health & Nutrition Letter* for their generous support of my books.

I am grateful to Robert Butler, M.D., and colleagues at the Brookdale Foundation for continuing encouragement of my efforts to bring solid science into the popular media.

This book has been enriched by the participation of men and women whose lives have been touched by osteoporosis. My warm thanks to Carol Quinlan, Isabel Chiang, and Jane Mosher for assisting with the illustrations, and to the women and men who shared their experiences and allowed us to tell their stories: Ann, Anne, Dorothy, Jill, Katie, Laura, Liz, Marie, Nan, Nancy, Pam, Sally, Sheila, Wendi, Dick, James, and Jerry. I've also benefited greatly from the support and comments of my Saturday morning workout group with my wonderful neighbors.

Finally, I want to express my love and gratitude to my dear family and friends. Once again they endured many days without me as I wrote this book—and encouraged me nonetheless.

Preface

◆ ◆ ◆

The past four years have been incredibly exciting for me. I never dreamed that so many women would be interested in strength training. Since the publication of my first book, *Strong Women Stay Young*, in 1997, I have received thousands of letters, e-mails, and phone calls from women all around the world who have been adventuresome enough to start strength training. I'm particularly delighted when I hear about generations of women exercising together—daughters, mothers, and sometimes grandmothers and great-grandmothers too.

As part of my mission to spread the word about strength training and women's health, I often speak to professional and community groups around the United States and abroad. Afterwards, I answer questions from the audience. Last year I noticed that more than half of these questions concerned osteoporosis. Increasingly, women know that it's so important to maintain their bones as they get older, but they're uncertain about the best strategy to follow. The answers involve nutrition and medication as well as exercise. I decided to write this book so I could pull together all the information women—and men—need to beat this terrible disease.

My research and the research of others have taught me a great deal about osteoporosis. But I've learned just as much from the women with whom I've worked. I know that the pain of osteoporosis is not just physical. This disease causes emotional pain and fear—changes that sap the vitality from too many women who still have meaningful lives to lead. I have seen personally how devastating it can be. The day I finished this book and sent it to my editor, my father called with bad news. His sister, one of my favorite aunts, who has suffered from osteoporosis for many years, had fallen and broken her hip and shoulder. This disease has destroyed her zest for life. Things would have been so different if the information and medication we have now had been available to her a decade ago.

Older women are taking steps to protect themselves from osteoporosis. Those who already have the disease are benefiting from new treatments. I'm also thrilled to see how many younger women are looking ahead and thinking about the problem too, because the sooner they begin preventive measures, the easier it is to maintain healthy bones.

I will turn 40 a month after this book is released. I'm more aware than ever that I'm at risk for this disease: I'm a woman; I'm white; I'm slender; and I have a family history of osteoporosis. And I'm also aware that I can take steps now to keep my bones strong for a lifetime. That's why no matter how busy I get, I work hard to maintain my active lifestyle and healthy diet.

Whatever your age, I urge you to heed this terrific slogan from the Massachusetts Osteoporosis Awareness Program:

Support your bones. They support you.

Osteoporosis
Is Preventable

CHAPTER 1

The Silent Crippler

◆ ◆ ◆

I do a lot of lectures at schools. I ask kids what someone with osteoporosis looks like, and they say, "An old lady all hunched over." Then I tell them that I have osteoporosis, and their jaws drop. I'm 34 and very athletic; I look like the picture of health. I tell them, "Don't take your bones for granted."

I was diagnosed at age 27. I was a competitive runner. I started having stress fractures in my feet and even in my femur. I broke my wrist three times—once I broke both of my wrists at the same time. I knew something wasn't right.

—JILL

Perhaps you have osteoporosis or bone loss already. Maybe you're wondering about your bones because your grandmother fractured her hip, or your mom is developing a "dowager's hump." You're wise to be concerned. Twenty-eight million Americans, mostly women, suffer from osteoporosis—dangerous thinning of the bones. When you have osteoporosis, your bones become so fragile they could break from a minor fall, from lifting a baby out of a crib, or even from an exuberant hug.

Though the obvious problems usually occur later in life, we now know that the invisible damage begins earlier—much earlier than most of us realize. For Jill, it probably started when she was in college. "I was a Division One track and cross-country runner on scholarship," she says. "My diet was well rounded but I was obsessive about exercise." A woman's estrogen levels can drop when she overexercises or undereats. One sign of low estrogen is missed periods. Jill didn't have regular menstrual periods for years.

Fortunately, most young women have normal cycles and enjoy the natural protection of estrogen, which plays a vital role in bone health. But as our estrogen production slows, bone loss begins. Starting around age 35 we lose up to 1 percent of our bone mass each year. These losses accelerate rapidly after menopause.

Osteoporosis is insidious because you can't see or feel what is happening. Most people who have the disease don't know it. And then a bone breaks. Each year 430,000 Americans wind up in the hospital because of fractures related to osteoporosis. Hip fractures—which represent about 300,000 of that total—are devastating. One victim in five dies within a year, and half are never able to live independently again. Most of us know someone who has suffered a hip fracture. But you may be surprised to learn that complications of this injury kill even more women every year than breast cancer. Preventing osteoporosis is really a life-and-death matter, like preventing cancer and heart disease.

Hip fractures are just the most obvious part of the problem. Millions of women suffer distressing symptoms that they don't connect to fragile bones. A woman may not realize that her chronic back pain comes from crush fractures in her spine. Fragile vertebras have crumbled under the ordinary stresses of everyday life. Osteoporosis can make a woman look old before her time—but she may have no idea that her slumped posture and protruding tummy are caused by fractures in her spine.

And then there's the emotional fallout. Katie, diagnosed with severe bone loss at age 54, fell into a deep depression:

> *I felt I didn't have a future. My mother had recently moved into a nursing home, and I thought, "I'll just take the next bed."*

> *I became a hermit. I was terrified of walking outdoors in the winter. If the street was slick with ice and I had to cross, I'd go up to a stranger and say, "Can I hold on to you—I'm afraid I'll fall." I quit walking at night. I quit carrying heavy groceries. I stopped walking the dog, because I was afraid she'd jerk the leash and I'd fall.*

With support from her husband, Katie began an exercise program and improved her diet; her doctor prescribed medication to help her bones. "It's still a challenge," says Katie, "but it feels really good to make my body stronger."

As a woman, you have one-in-three odds of suffering from osteoporosis in your lifetime. But you can beat those odds. Medical experts now consider osteoporosis a preventable disease. And it's treatable. Thanks to new findings about nutrition and exercise, as well as new medications, you can protect yourself—provided you know how.

Sheila

February: "I'm too young to feel this old."

The first time Sheila wrote to me, she described herself as age "44 going on 60." The previous year she'd been diagnosed with osteoporosis. She wrote:

I am tired and weak. My body is very flabby and I'm ashamed to wear shorts or sleeveless shirts. I am feeling very discouraged.

March: "I've joined a strength-training class."

A month later, Sheila e-mailed again to say she'd begun strength training:

I'm gradually adding more weight to my program and have more energy. The class has boosted my confidence. I also purchased a yoga video and my balance and flexibility have improved.

July: "They call me Tool Time Momma."

Sheila's latest report:

There's such a big difference, and it's not all physical. I feel stronger emotionally too. I just returned from a church project in Alaska. We built a parsonage for a mission church. They had a kitchen crew that fed everyone—most of the women worked on that—and a construction crew. I was on the construction crew. The other people on the crew, mostly men, were surprised to see what I could lift. They started calling me Tool Time Momma. On the last night of the project, they gave me an award.

MYTHS ABOUT OSTEOPOROSIS

Some women don't give a thought to osteoporosis—even though they really should. Others are terrified, but uncertain about what to do. Or they may *think* they're doing everything possible to prevent osteoporosis. They diligently exercise and carefully watch their diet—but the measures they've adopted are not the most effective ones.

◆ ◆ ◆

I took a bone density test four years ago, and it found just a slight degree of osteoporosis. Even that shocked me. I was 61, but for years I had been running about 20 miles a week and eating right. I was so sure that my diet and running program were keeping my bones healthy. My doctor pointed out that if I weren't doing the things I was doing, it might have been worse.

—SALLY

◆ ◆ ◆

Do you still believe these common myths about osteoporosis?

Myth #1: Osteoporosis is an old lady's disease.

Women in their twenties and thirties can get osteoporosis. Fortunately, this doesn't happen often; most early victims of the disease have significant risk factors such as prolonged use of steroid medications or lengthy periods of eating disorders. Ironically, many of these women are dancers or athletes, who look healthy and fit.

The bones we have later in life reflect what we did as kids, teens, and young adults. So in a very real sense, osteoporosis is a disease that starts in childhood.

◆ ◆ ◆

I'm 44 and I was diagnosed with osteoporosis last year. But in retrospect, I'm sure I've had it since my thirties, because I had an eating disorder for many years. I feel different. Only my two best friends know I have osteoporosis. Most people would wonder why it's so bad in a woman my age, and it's embarrassing to admit what I did to myself. My mother's bones are better than mine. She's always taken good care of herself, and it's paying off.

—LAURA

◆ ◆ ◆

Myth #2: After menopause, women can prevent osteoporosis by consuming calcium-fortified foods and beverages and taking calcium supplements.

Many women religiously drink milk, buy calcium-fortified cereal, and take a calcium supplement just to be sure. If women are premenopausal, extra calcium can help build strong bones. But simply upping calcium consumption has *never* been shown to increase bone density or prevent fractures in older women. Add vitamin D to that calcium, and the effects are dramatic: bone density increases significantly and fractures are reduced by 50 percent. That's because vitamin D is needed to absorb calcium and turn it into bone, and many postmenopausal women don't get enough. New research suggests that other nutrients are important too.

Myth #3: Walking is the best exercise for preventing and treating osteoporosis.

Walking is a wonderful exercise—for the heart. But no study has ever shown that a middle-aged or older woman can increase her bone density by taking up walking. The light impact of walking provides only mild stimulation to bone. If you've been walking for *decades,* that can add up. Women with a lifelong habit of regular walking have higher bone density—and a 30 percent lower fracture rate—than their sedentary age-mates. However, the short-term effects of walking on bone are minor. Even a yearlong walking program has very little effect.

Please don't think I'm criticizing walking! On the contrary, it's one of my favorite physical activities. There's no other aerobic exercise that's as easy to tuck into a busy schedule. And it's safe for nearly everyone. I strongly encourage you to develop a walking habit—it will help retard further bone loss and has many other health benefits. Similarly, swimming and bike riding are terrific exercises for the heart. But because they're low-impact and don't involve weight bearing, they do very little for your bones. Again, I'm not suggesting you give up these enjoyable activities. But if you want to prevent osteoporosis and fractures, your exercise program should include more.

As you probably know by now, weight lifting isn't just for people who want to look like Ms. Olympia or Arnold Schwarzenegger. My research and numerous other investigations have shown that with just two or three strength-training sessions per week, women can halt bone loss and even regain bone density. And they do *not* develop bulky muscles! On the contrary, they usually become trimmer and shapelier.

We're also learning that higher-impact aerobic activities, such as jumping and stair climbing, can be very helpful for bone—provided they're done carefully. Also very important is balance training to prevent falls. Think about it: If your bones are fragile, the last thing you want is to fall. Our balancing ability usually declines with age, so falling becomes a significant risk. A program combining exercises that improve both bone density and balance can dramatically reduce your risk of fractures from osteoporosis.

ABOUT THE RESEARCH

Searching for the best bone-boosting exercise

Back in the mid-1980s, I recruited thirty-six sedentary women ages 50 to 70 to see if an ambitious walking program would help their bones. We gave the women bone density tests, then divided them into two groups. Half the women met four times a week for a year and spent fifty minutes walking. The others—the control group—simply remained sedentary.

Our laboratory is in downtown Boston, near the Boston Common and the Public Gardens—perfect spots for walking. I walked with the women in my study, and we had a great time. After a year, we measured the women's bone density again. What a disappointment! Walking had no effect at all on bone density in the hip. There was a slight benefit to the spine: the walkers maintained their bone density, while the controls lost bone in their spine.

Meanwhile, my colleagues at Tufts were exploring the effects of strength training. Intrigued by their findings, I began another study of postmenopausal women. This time, those in the exercise group came to the laboratory twice a week and lifted weights. One year later, the volunteers in our control group, the ones who didn't exercise, had lost about 2 percent of their bone density. That's not unusual for women after menopause. But the women who strength-trained actually *gained* an average of 1 percent. What's more, their scores on a balance test increased by 14 percent, further reducing their risk of fractures. These findings were published in the *Journal of the American Medical Association* in 1994.

Myth #4: Once you've lost bone, you can never get it back.

The latest treatments can actually restore bone. I'm not saying that a woman with osteoporosis can recover all the bone she's lost—we don't yet have treatments that effective. But even small gains in bone density can make a meaningful difference in the chances of a fracture. Hormone replacement therapy and newer medications can reduce the odds by an astonishing 50 to 75 percent. And there's evidence that a combination of medication, exercise, and nutritional measures is even more effective.

◆ ◆ ◆

I'm 48 and I've taken Synthroid for a thyroid condition for many years. I know that can affect bones, so I've been concerned. I talked to my doctor about two years ago, and she said it would be a good idea for me to have a baseline bone density test. It was normal.

There's a lot we can't control, but I tend to be a person who seeks out ways to have control over my future. I was already doing aerobic exercise— mostly riding a bike and sometimes swimming laps. I decided to switch to weight-bearing exercise because of my bones. Now I nearly always jog, walk, or use a stair-climbing machine. I started to take calcium and vitamin D, and to work hard to have three to four dairy portions per day. I also began weight lifting twice a week.

A few months ago I had the bone density test redone. It showed a 5 percent gain in bone mass.

—PAM

◆ ◆ ◆

Myth #5: Men can't get osteoporosis.

Alas, they can. An estimated two million men have this disease, which is tragically undertreated in men. A man is far more likely to suffer an osteoporosis-related fracture during his lifetime than he is to get prostate can-

James

I'm a radiologist. Last year we were checking out a new bone density–testing machine. I hopped up on the machine myself to see what being tested was like. My results were grossly abnormal, indicating osteoporosis. That seemed impossible. I was a 37-year-old man in excellent health. I assumed the machine was defective. But I tested myself on different equipment and the same numbers came up.

Though I was shocked by the diagnosis, it explained several puzzling fractures. Six months earlier, on a trip to the lake with my family, I'd broken three ribs falling into the water. I thought it was just bad luck. The year before, I'd slipped on an icy patch in the parking lot and fractured my shoulder blade. My orthopedist had been puzzled. He looked at the X ray and said, "I'm surprised you didn't just dislocate the shoulder. It's unusual to have a fracture from that trauma." But I'd been carrying heavy packages, so I figured I must have fallen in a funny way. Neither of us thought of osteoporosis. But after the test, I understood why my bones had broken so easily.

I had no obvious risk factors. I was physically fit and very active—I'm the captain of a bicycling team; my diet was good. My primary-care doctor gave me a full physical, and I learned I had an endocrine problem: low testosterone. As I read more, I realized I'd been showing symptoms of a deficiency for some time. My energy had been low and I hadn't felt right. I'd been wondering if it was just middle age.

I take testosterone, Fosamax, and calcium supplements with vitamin D. I use a treadmill; I started weight training. I love it. Being stronger is very satisfying. I've been on this therapy for sixteen months, and I feel terrific. In less than two years my bone density has increased to a point where I no longer have a diagnosis of osteoporosis.

cer. Yet men—and even their doctors—are largely unaware of the problem. A Gallup survey of men found that fewer than 2 percent had been told by their doctor that they may be at risk for osteoporosis. This book is written mainly for women, but men can follow the program and help their bones too—a special just-for-men chapter explains how.

THE *STRONG WOMEN, STRONG BONES* PROGRAM

No matter what your age, no matter what your starting point, this program will help you improve your bones. Even if you've already had significant bone loss or fractures, it's not too late.

The *Strong Women, Strong Bones* program combines the three essential measures for preventing and treating osteoporosis: nutrition, physical activity, and (when appropriate) medication. I want to emphasize that these elements work most powerfully when used together. For instance, if you're already taking hormone replacement therapy, you can further reduce your risk of fractures by doing strength training as well.

Nutrition

You probably watch your diet, but it might need minor adjustments for optimal bone benefits. Most women find that when they make changes for the sake of their bones, they end up eating better for overall health.

Calcium gets all the attention, but it's just one of the key nutrients for healthy bones. Vitamin D is essential—perhaps even more important than calcium. The best diet for bones also includes plenty of fruits and vegetables. We now know that the nutrients responsible for this benefit include vitamin K, vitamin C, magnesium, potassium, and possibly other vitamins and minerals. And we're beginning to suspect that soy has special promise for bone too.

Physical activity

I hope you're already physically active. If so, you can continue the exercise you enjoy. But you may not be doing everything possible for strong bones. This book will help you fill in the gaps. And if you're currently sedentary, the program will ease you into a more active, healthier lifestyle.

Exciting new research shows that just two minutes a day of vertical jumping—yes, leaping up and down—can produce significant improvements in bone. I know you've heard warnings about the dangers of high-impact activities for joints, and of course, jumping isn't appropriate for everyone. But healthy, fit women under age 50 can benefit from jumping if they follow appropriate cautions. And different higher-impact activities, such as stair climbing, are safe for most women. The *Strong Women, Strong Bones* program includes vertical jumping where appropriate, plus a combination of other exercises that have proven value for bone.

Medication

If you're like me, you'd probably rather not take medication. But this is a very beneficial part of treatment for women with bone loss. Until just a short time ago, options were quite limited. But several powerful new medications have changed that. One new drug not only builds bone—it also decreases the risk of breast cancer.

HOW THIS BOOK WILL HELP YOU

It's easy to take our bones for granted, especially when we're young and menopause seems far away. But our skeleton has to last a lifetime. *Strong Women, Strong Bones* will give you all the information you need to take charge of your bone health.

Here's what the book contains:

The latest scientific information

Women tell me that they're more motivated to make lifestyle changes when they understand the reasons behind them. This is especially important for a disease like osteoporosis, which advances invisibly. Symptoms rarely appear until bone loss has become significant. So you need to know what's happening under the skin before it's too late.

- Chapter 2 describes the process by which bone is formed—and the many factors that influence that process.
- Chapter 3 explains how osteoporosis develops, and tells you the earliest signs to watch for.

The essential tests

We're much more fortunate than our mothers and grandmothers. Osteoporosis struck earlier generations of women without warning. But we have resources that can alert us to the danger long before we fracture a bone.

- Chapter 4 will help you figure out if you're at special risk for bone loss.
- Chapter 5 explains how bone density testing works and why this exam is every bit as important as regular mammograms. The best bone density tests predict fractures more successfully than cholesterol levels predict heart attacks or blood pressure predicts stroke. Yet these tests are underutilized, and insurance doesn't always cover them. As a result, less than 10 percent of people with significant bone loss are aware of their problem. You'll find out if you need to be tested, and you'll learn how to make your case with your HMO or insurance company.
- Chapter 6 looks at a forgotten factor in osteoporosis: falls. You may be surprised when you take the balance tests in this chapter! Poor balance isn't just a problem of the elderly. Most of us begin to lose our balancing ability well before age 50. Fortunately, there's a lot you can do to protect yourself, from simple balance exercises to fall-proofing your home.

A plan for action

The next three chapters get down to work.

- Chapter 7 helps you evaluate your diet and make changes. The chapter includes five complete daily menus, showing how anyone can follow a bone-boosting diet—even women who are watching their weight or who don't eat dairy products.
- Chapter 8 provides complete instructions for a comprehensive exercise program designed to strengthen your bones. The program features weight-bearing aerobic exercise, strength training, vertical jumping (if appropriate), balance exercises, and stretching. That

might sound like a lot, but once you master the moves, they take less than three hours a week. You'll learn how to devise customized workouts that are safe, effective, and convenient.

- Chapter 9 describes all currently approved medications for preventing and treating osteoporosis, including hormone replacement therapy, Fosamax, Evista, and calcitonin. No single option is right for everyone. I'll also discuss many unproven treatments that women have questions about.

- Chapter 10 is a mini-workbook that will help you pull everything together. I'll walk you through a one-hour-per-year plan for setting goals and staying on track.

◆　◆　◆

I started hormone replacement therapy, and I began strength training. The next year I took the bone density test again and did better.

At this point I'm lifting weights, running, walking, hiking, and cycling. I run up and down the two flights of stairs in my house a million times a day. I'm drinking calcium-fortified orange juice; eating other good stuff, like low-fat dairy products and canned salmon complete with bones; taking calcium supplements plus a multivitamin with Vitamin D; continuing with hormone replacement—and not worrying.

—SALLY, AGE 65

◆　◆　◆

Also included:

The book has these additional features:

- Chapter 11 discusses osteoporosis in men, and explains how men can adapt the program in this book.
- Chapter 12 provides answers to frequently asked questions.
- Appendices include a glossary and a bibliography.

Osteoporosis is *not* an inevitable part of getting older. The *Strong Women, Strong Bones* program is designed to prevent bone loss and fractures. But it does so much more than that. The same measures that help your bones also improve your health—and your emotional well-being—in many other ways.

Anne

Three years ago, I fell on stairs at an appliance store. I crashed down and broke my left wrist so badly I was hospitalized. They tested my bones, and I was diagnosed with osteoporosis. I began exercising. Three times a week I go to a fitness center. I lift heavy weights, walk and run on a treadmill, and use a stair climber. I also started taking medication. The following year I fell and broke my wrist again, but that time the break was milder. And last year I had two falls and didn't break anything.

I used to love climbing in the White Mountains, but I'd stopped. Now I can do it again. It's like I've gotten a little younger. This summer I backpacked in Yosemite with my oldest son and my granddaughter. We camped out in back country for seven days and six nights. I carried a 30-pound pack with no problems. I had a lot of joy on this trip. We climbed the Half Dome at Yosemite. It's quite a place. The trail is just a narrow ledge carved into the rock. A man climbing ahead of us heard my son call me Mom. He turned around and asked me, "How old are you?" I told him, "I'm 74." He almost fell off the mountain.

CHAPTER 2

The Secret Life
of Bone

◆ ◆ ◆

O ur bodies contain over two hundred bones, but we can't see them. Press a finger to your forearm or hip, and explore your bones through your skin. They feel hard, more like stone than like flesh. Indeed, the word "skeleton" comes from the Greek *skeletos,* which means "dried up." But bone is very much alive. Like all living tissue, it constantly repairs and renews itself. And it needs our nurturing to remain in good health.

Bones serve three important functions, two of which you'd probably guess. First, the skeleton gives structure to our bodies, allowing us to stand upright and move. Without our bones we'd collapse, like a tent without poles. Bones also protect our fragile internal organs. The skull encases the brain; the ribs shelter the heart; the vertebras protect the spinal cord. Bone has a third function that's less obvious, but just as vital: it serves as a warehouse of essential minerals, especially calcium.

This chapter takes you under the skin, and explains the surprisingly complex activities of bone. When you understand the basics, you'll be ready to learn how osteoporosis develops and why various treatments work.

BENEATH THE SURFACE

W hat you feel when you touch your bones through skin is just their outer shell. Underneath is a more porous layer, with a honeycomb structure. Though both layers are called "bone," and both are hard, they're actually two different kinds of tissue:

- **Cortical** or dense bone, the outer layer, is very compact and heavy. About 80 percent of our bone mass is cortical bone.
- **Trabecular** or spongy bone, the porous inner layer, is light and has a lattice structure. Approximately 20 percent of our bone mass is trabecular bone.

As you might guess from looking at the picture below, cortical bone is considerably stronger than trabecular bone. All our bones contain both types, but the proportion varies. The long bones of our arms and legs consist mainly of hard cortical bone, though the ends are mostly the spongy trabecular type. Other bones—including the vertebras of the spine, the small bones of the wrist, and the pelvis—are trabecular, with just a thin outer shell of cortical bone. Trabecular bone is especially vulnerable to osteoporosis. That's why so many osteoporotic fractures occur in the spine, the wrist, and the hip—these areas include significant amounts of trabecular bone.

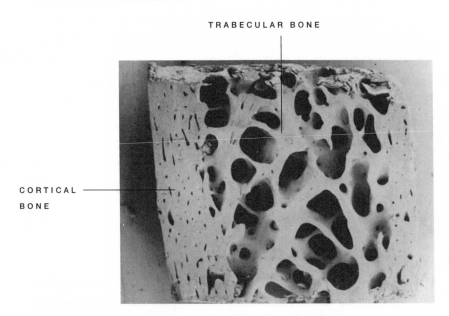

TRABECULAR BONE

CORTICAL
BONE

Structure of cortical bone and trabecular bone

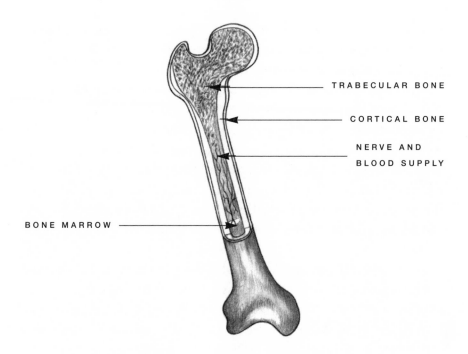

TRABECULAR BONE

CORTICAL BONE

NERVE AND
BLOOD SUPPLY

BONE MARROW

Inside a thigh bone

Under the hard outer layer of cortical bone is the honeycomb trabecular bone. In the middle of its length, the bone is mostly cortical; toward both ends, it's mainly trabecular. Blood vessels and nerves run through bone tissue. In the center is a hollow channel that contains bone marrow, which manufactures blood cells.

HOW BONE IS MADE

If you could look at your skeleton under a powerful microscope, you'd see something that resembles a construction site swarming with busy "crews" of bone cells. As one crew demolishes a small area of bone, another arrives to rebuild it. The health of our bones depends upon this process, which is called **remodeling.**

The bone cells responsible for demolition are the **osteoclasts.** They secrete an acid that dissolves old bone. As they work, calcium and other minerals are released from the dissolved bone into the bloodstream. Most of this material is recycled later in the remodeling process. But some is used for other functions, as I'll explain shortly. It's important to realize that whenever your body needs extra calcium, it signals the osteoclasts to dissolve more bone. That's why it's so important to consume enough.

The osteoclasts dissolve enough bone to create a tiny cavity. As they finish their work, they die and the second stage of remodeling begins. A crew of different cells—the **osteoblasts**—assembles at the site. They line the cavity with collagen, the soft, sticky substance that forms the framework for bone. Then they draw calcium and other minerals from the blood, forming crystals on the collagen. The collagen and minerals harden into bone tissue. As the osteoblasts finish their work, they're transformed into mature bone cells and become part of the new bone. They're still alive, but they're no longer active.

At the end of the remodeling cycle, the cavity has been refilled with new bone. The whole process takes three to six months—far longer than renewal of other body tissues. That's why broken bones heal so much more slowly than injuries to the skin or muscles. And that's why osteoporosis treatments and preventive measures take a long time to show effects.

Terminology tip

Here's a simple way to remember which type of bone cell is which:

Osteo*c*lasts *c*lear away bone.
Osteo*b*lasts *b*uild bone.

When the osteoclasts are more active than osteoblasts, the dissolving stage of remodeling gets ahead of the rebuilding phase. The result is loss of bone.

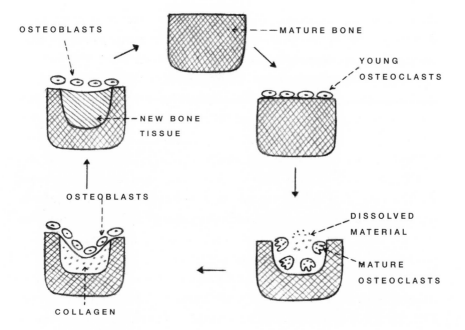

Bone remodeling

1. *Remodeling begins when young osteoclasts arrive at the site.*
2. *Mature osteoclasts dissolve old bone, creating a cavity.*
3. *Osteoblasts line the cavity with collagen.*
4. *Crystals of calcium and other minerals are drawn into the collagen, forming new bone tissue.*
5. *The cavity is filled, and the remodeling cycle is complete.*

THE THREE MAJOR FACTORS THAT DETERMINE BONE MASS

Our bones grow slowly, and their density reflects our entire life history. Three factors are most responsible for shaping our skeletons:

#1: Estrogen

Because estrogen is a sex hormone, many women don't realize that most tissues in the body—even ones like bone that don't seem related to sex—have special receptors for estrogen. That's why menopause affects so much more than the menstrual cycle. Throughout our lives, bone mass rises and falls along with our estrogen levels.

Estrogen stimulates the bone-building activity of the osteoblasts. Even more important, it suppresses the bone-dissolving activity of the osteoclasts. After menopause, the brakes let up. The main reason we lose bone during normal aging isn't that the osteoblasts stop building; it's that their efforts are outdone by the out-of-control osteoclasts.

Estrogen also has indirect effects on bone. Bone-building cells have more available calcium before menopause because estrogen helps the intestines absorb calcium from food and also promotes conservation of calcium by the kidneys, so less is excreted. In addition, estrogen stimulates activity of vitamin D, which is essential for calcium metabolism.

Other hormones also affect bone—including calcitonin, growth hormone, parathyroid hormone, and testosterone. (Yes, women produce small amounts of testosterone too.) Yet another indirect effect of estrogen is that it helps regulate release of these other hormones. You'll hear more about these complicated processes when I discuss medication in Chapter 9.

Can chronic stress or depression harm bones?

It's easy to imagine that a woman who has osteoporosis might become anxious or depressed. But could anxiety or depression actually *cause* bone loss? That was the surprising finding of a 1996 study published in the *New England Journal of Medicine*. The subjects were twenty-four pairs of women ages 30 to 40. The women were matched for weight and nutritional status, but one member of each pair had a long history of depression while the other did not. The investigators found that those who were depressed had lower bone density.

What's the explanation? We're not yet sure, but it could be related to cortisol, a hormone released when a person is under stress. Cortisol, which is produced by the adrenal gland, suppresses bone formation and also decreases calcium absorption—two effects that are detrimental to bone.

#2: Physical activity

We've known for centuries that when body tissues are used, they adapt to the challenge. If we lift weights, our muscles get stronger. If we run or engage in other vigorous aerobic activities, the capability of our heart and lungs increases. As early as the late nineteenth century, scientists hypothesized that bone responded similarly. But they didn't have any way to measure bone density in living people.

Additional insights came in the 1940s and 1950s from fascinating studies of bed rest. Doctors and nurses had noticed, to their dismay, that hospital patients often grew weaker as they recovered from an illness or surgery. They guessed that bedridden patients were losing muscle and bone. When investigators followed these patients closely, they discovered that after just one week of bed rest, calcium levels in the urine increased dramatically. Inactivity actually dissolved bones!

Studies of returning astronauts in the 1960s (see box) confirmed this finding. Researchers also learned that bone was regained once patients became active again. Standard medical practices eventually changed as a result of this work. If you've been hospitalized recently, you know that patients are encouraged to get on their feet as quickly as possible, even after major surgery.

Warning: Space travel may be harmful to your bones!

In the early days of the space program, returning astronauts were so weak that sometimes they had to be carried out of their flight capsules. Tests revealed that they'd lost both muscle and bone. These healthy, vigorous men dropped an average 1 percent of their bone mass in just a week. One reason: weightlessness.

These startling findings showed how much our bones need the challenge of gravity. These days, astronauts exercise on special machines that allow them to work their muscles. They still suffer some bone loss, because workouts only partly compensate for the lack of gravity, but the effects are less severe.

In the late 1960s and 1970s, scientists finally devised practical tools for measuring bone density. This inspired a wave of research on bone development and physical activity. Though we now know how bone responds to physical activity, we're still not sure exactly why it happens. But at least three mechanisms are involved:

- Bone-building osteoblasts are stimulated by the mechanical forces that exercise generates. Each time your feet hit the ground when you're walking, your bones are stimulated to grow. That's why walking is better for bones than swimming, and why jogging and running—which are higher-impact activities—are better than walking.
- The chronic force of muscles pulling against bones also promotes osteoblast activity. The stronger your muscles, the more stimulation they give to your bones. You don't notice this stimulation as much as you'd notice the impact of running and other weight-bearing activities. But because it's happening constantly, the effect on bone is very powerful.
- Physical activity increases secretion of growth hormone, as well as other hormones that encourage bone and muscle growth. You'll have higher levels of these hormones if you get plenty of exercise.

We see these mechanisms at work in studies of elite athletes. For example, one investigation compared the left and right arms of professional tennis players. The bones in their racket arm were 15 to 20 percent denser than bones in the other arm. Another investigation, which measured the leg bones of cross-country runners and those of nonrunners the same age, found that the runners' bones were 10 to 20 percent denser. More recent studies have shown that men and women who lift weights have spine and hip bones about 10 percent denser than those of runners. The lesson for all of us: The more stimulation our bones receive from our muscles and the impact of exercise, the denser they will be.

#3: Nutrition

Good nutrition is essential to strong bones. As we get older, a healthy diet becomes even more important: we're at greater risk for losing bone, and our bodies don't process nutrients as efficiently. The two most important nutrients for bone are calcium and vitamin D. But in the past decade we've learned that other minerals and vitamins play significant roles too. As you'll see, most of these nutrients come from fruits and vegetables. We also know from population studies that people who eat plenty of fruits and vegetables—especially soy—have better bone health. But we don't yet know all the reasons why. Research is exploding in this area, and we're beginning to get answers.

ABOUT THE SCIENCE

Why fruits and vegetables are good for bones

Back in 1968, an article published in the medical journal *Lancet* hypothesized that a diet with less meat and more fruits and vegetables would result in better bones. The reason: a better balance of acid in the blood.

Our bodies work hard to maintain just the right level of acidity in our blood. One mechanism for correcting an excess is to dissolve some bone, releasing acid-neutralizing minerals—potassium, magnesium, and calcium. In effect, our skeleton is like a large antacid tablet. Indeed, some antacids contain those very same minerals.

Interest in the acid hypothesis continues to this day. Katherine Tucker, Ph.D., along with other colleagues at Tufts, followed 1,164 men and women who participated in the famed Framingham Heart study. The investigators looked at the volunteers' food intake and gave them bone density tests. The results, published in 1999 in the *American Journal of Clinical Nutrition*, showed a strong positive correlation between fruit and vegetable intake and bone-mineral density.

Minerals

Minerals are the substance from which our skeleton is formed. Our bones are about 38 percent calcium. But calcium isn't the only mineral in bone. About 17 percent of bone mass is phosphorus. Bones also contain magnesium, potassium, zinc, and sodium.

Most of us have no difficulty consuming healthy amounts of all these essential minerals—except for calcium. Ninety percent of American women don't get as much calcium as they need from the foods they eat. Fortunately, the problem is easily corrected. In Chapter 7 I'll help you figure out if you're consuming enough calcium, and explain what to do if you're not.

Vitamins

Vitamins play a different but equally essential role. They're necessary catalysts in various biochemical reactions involved in bone formation. We've known since the 1920s that Vitamin D is required for calcium absorption—without it, our body can't use the calcium we consume. This crucial vitamin also helps the osteoblasts incorporate minerals into bone. We now know that other vitamins are needed for bone development as well. For instance, vitamins C and K contribute in different ways to collagen production, the first stage of bone formation.

The surprising seasons of bone density

Unless we take vitamin D supplements, our bones change with the seasons, reflecting our exposure to the vitamin D–forming rays of the sun. Bone density reaches its annual peak after the summer. Seasonal losses begin later in the fall as the days get shorter. We reach our annual low in late spring. And then the days grow longer again. The difference between high and low points can amount to 3 to 4 percent. That's why it's very important to consistently schedule bone density tests for the same time of year.

CALCIUM IS CRUCIAL!

Calcium is necessary for more than bone. It plays an essential role in vital functions, including transmission of nerve impulses, blood coagulation, regulation of blood pressure, and muscle contractions. Every time our heart beats, every time we lift a finger or blink an eye, calcium is used. We get this calcium from two sources: the food we consume and our bones.

Our body regulates calcium very closely, with an intricate system of interrelated mechanisms that constantly inch our blood calcium level up or down to keep it in the narrow optimal range. If we get plenty of calcium in our diet, we don't have to draw down the supply that's stored in our skeleton. But if there's a chronic insufficiency, our body will sacrifice our bones to obtain the calcium it needs. Some medications used to prevent and treat osteoporosis are based on our understanding of calcium regulation.

When the body needs more calcium

A drop in blood calcium levels triggers several mechanisms that bring it back up. These are subtle adjustments, like your tiny turns of the steering wheel when you're driving down a straight highway.

- Secretion of parathyroid hormone is increased. The parathyroid glands—four tiny glands in the neck—promote activity of the osteoclasts. As these cells dissolve bone, calcium is released into the blood.
- Additional vitamin D is converted to its active form by the kidneys. This increases absorption of calcium from food. Ordinarily, our body absorbs only about 20 to 35 percent of our calcium intake, but this can rise significantly if necessary.
- Kidneys begin conserving calcium, excreting less of it in the urine.

BONE DEVELOPMENT THROUGH LIFE

Our skeleton is like a bank account. The more we deposit in our early working years—and the more carefully we spend—the more comfortable our cushion will be later in life when we retire.

For the first twenty-five years of life, our bodies are programmed to add bone. How much we accumulate depends on our sex (men add more, thanks to testosterone), our genes, our health, and our lifestyle, especially diet and exercise. This early period is so important to future bone health that some experts refer to osteoporosis as a pediatric disease with geriatric outcomes.

In the second half of life, our natural tendency is to lose bone. Nevertheless, there's a great deal we can do to prevent or at least retard those losses.

Childhood

Thanks to growth hormone, which stimulates the construction work of the osteoblasts, bones grow dramatically during childhood. From birth to age 2, bone mass doubles. By age 10, it has doubled again.

Adolescence

Bone growth accelerates at puberty, when sex hormones begin to work their magic. Youngsters may grow 4 to 6 inches in a single year; their bones become longer and thicker. By the time puberty is over, teens typically have double the bone mass they had at age 10.

We can add bone at any time of life, but never as easily as during adolescence, when the body is designed to grow. These are also the years when lifelong habits are formed, and those affect bone as well. By age 18 we've accumulated about 90 percent of the bone mass we'll have at our maximum.

Young adulthood

Bone continues to develop after adolescence, but at a much slower rate. Most of us slowly reach our peak bone mass in our early to mid twenties. Through our early thirties, the bone remodeling process that I explained earlier is just about in balance: our bodies build approximately as much bone as they lose.

Some women experience unusually early or rapid bone loss. In fact, women in their twenties can lose significant amounts of bone if they have eating disorders, menstrual irregularities, or other medical problems. (In Chapter 4 I'll discuss these and other risk factors.)

◆ ◆ ◆

I had an eating disorder off and on for years, starting in my twenties. At one point I weighed 78 pounds. My periods stopped. A psychiatrist told me I might get osteoporosis, but I dismissed it. I figured I'd just go on estrogen after menopause. Then last year I turned my left foot while I was jogging, and I broke a metatarsal bone. The doctor checked it every two weeks, but it didn't heal. This went on for three months. I told him about my past history, and said I was concerned that I'd damaged my bones. The doctor said I couldn't have osteoporosis at my age—I was 43—but he reluctantly gave me a test. I had severe osteoporosis.

—LAURA

◆ ◆ ◆

Bone during pregnancy and lactation

Pregnancy and breast-feeding place extra demands on a woman's body. Hormonal changes enable her system to use calcium much more efficiently, but this doesn't fully compensate. So it's essential for expectant moms to increase their calcium intake and eat well. This is especially important for women who breast-feed their babies for more than six months, or who have closely spaced pregnancies. With a good diet, a new mother can probably restore lost bone within a year after she stops nursing.

The premenopausal years

In our mid-thirties our bones reach a turning point. The balance between the osteoclasts and the osteoblasts begins to shift, and for the first time in our lives we lose more bone than we build. Each year during this premenopausal period, our bone mass decreases by half a percent to 1 percent.

Declining estrogen production is the main reason for this change, but it's not the only factor. As we get older, our bodies become less able to absorb calcium from the food we eat, at least in part because our skin produces less vitamin D.

Most of us still have an ample margin of safety during these years, so bone loss doesn't yet make us vulnerable to fractures. But the more bone mass we can preserve at this stage, the better prepared we are for the future.

Menopause

During the year or two before menopause and the first five years afterwards, when estrogen levels drop, we experience a dramatic change in bone. Without estrogen to contain them, the bone-dissolving osteoclasts increase their activity by about 20 percent; the osteoblasts don't increase to match. The net effect is loss of bone. Menopausal women typically lose 1 to 3 percent of their bone mass annually, and some lose as much as 5 percent. Because change is so rapid, these years are a critical time for preventive measures.

Five years postmenopause to age 70

The rate of bone loss slows down, but it's still about 1 to 2 percent per year. During these years, when the average woman has only 60 to 70 percent of her peak bone mass, the skeleton may become dangerously fragile.

Age 70 and older

Fortunately, the rate of loss declines further, to less than half a percent to 1 percent per year. But many women have lost so much bone by this time that any additional loss significantly increases their risk of fractures. By age 85 or 90, a woman may have only half the bone mass she had at her peak.

Many factors affect our bone mass, only some of which we can control—and nature isn't always in our favor. But bone remains dynamic through our entire life. At any age we can reduce the risk of osteoporosis and fractures. Moreover, exciting new evidence suggests we can even *add* bone. It's never too late to make a difference!

The Anatomy of Osteoporosis

◆ ◆ ◆

Osteoporosis is a silent disease. You can lose bone for years and not realize it—until you fall. The physical discomfort of other chronic diseases is no fun, but at least it sounds the alarm. The tragedy of osteoporosis is that there are no early symptoms: you don't feel any different; there's no pain or any outward sign. So it often strikes without warning, when bone loss is already advanced.

An osteoporotic fracture isn't like breaking your arm in junior high, when you spend a few weeks in a cast covered with your friends' scribbles, then emerge as good as new. After bones heal, you may be left with pain and deformities. Your life may be changed—not only by disability but also by the fear and depression that so often afflict those who suffer from osteoporosis.

This chapter sheds light on the invisible process of bone loss. The very good news is that osteoporosis is now a preventable disease—if you start early enough. And if you already have osteoporosis, it *is* treatable.

SILENT SABOTAGE

Most scientists believe that some bone loss is inevitable with age. But if we take steps to minimize the losses, we can keep our bones out of the fracture zone. Thanks to new tests, described in Chapter 5, you can learn if your bones are dangerously weak.

Doctors differentiate between two degrees of bone loss:

- **Osteopenia,** which is abnormally low bone density, and
- **Osteoporosis,** a more severe condition in which so much bone has been lost that bone tissue is literally porous—hence the word "osteoporosis."

As osteopenia advances to osteoporosis, the microarchitecture of bone tissue deteriorates. Bones become much weaker, and the risk of fractures rises. Bone density is the single best predictor of future fractures. If you look at the pictures—which show microscopic views of bone—you'll understand why.

◆　◆　◆

When you don't need to know about osteoporosis, you think it's just about stooped shoulders. It doesn't seem a big deal. But then you find out from people who have it.

—ANN

◆　◆　◆

THE VULNERABLE BONES

When bone density is low, any bone in the body is much more likely to fracture. But a combination of factors make the spine, wrist, and hip bones especially vulnerable.

The spine

The delicate bones of the spine—the vertebras—consist mostly of trabecular bone tissue. Because of their small size and fragile structure, vertebras become extremely susceptible to fractures when bone mass is lost. If a woman has osteoporosis, vertebras can be fractured by everyday activities—picking up a suitcase, sneezing, or bending down to tie her shoelaces.

Vertebral fractures are the most common kind that result from osteo-

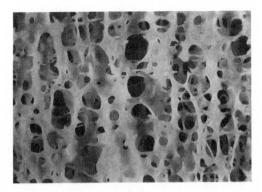

Microscopic view of normal bone

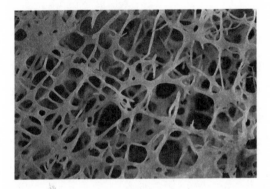

Microscopic view of bone with osteopenia

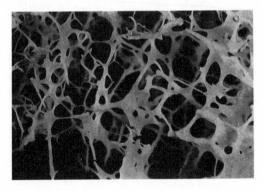

Microscopic view of bone with osteoporosis

porosis. An estimated 700,000 spinal fractures occur each year in the United States. About a third of women over age 60—and half of women over 80—have at least one vertebral fracture. High as these numbers are, they may underestimate the problem, because as many as two out of three vertebral fractures are never diagnosed.

It might seem odd that a woman could fracture her spine and not know. But only half of vertebral fractures are associated with falls, and they don't always cause pain. A woman with severe osteoporosis can fracture her spine just by bending forward. If she feels pain, she might assume she'd simply strained a muscle in her back.

A guide to your spine

Your spine consists of twenty-four vertebras plus a larger flat bone at the bottom, the sacrum, and a tiny tailbone underneath, which is the coccyx. You can feel your vertebras—the line of little bumps down the center of your back. To cushion the vertebras as you move, a flat cylindrical disk, made from tough cartilage, lies between each pair.

The spine is divided into three sections:

- **The cervical spine** includes the top seven vertebras. This section of the spine supports the head. It's the least likely to fracture from osteoporosis.
- **The thoracic spine** consists of the twelve vertebras that run down the back of the chest, each attached to a pair of ribs. This is the area where most osteoporotic fractures occur. The characteristic bent-over posture of osteoporosis results from fractures in the thoracic spine.
- **The lumbar spine** has five vertebras. Pain in the lumbar spine can result from fractures or from other problems.

Symptoms

As you read this chapter, you may recognize certain symptoms. If so, it's important to find out whether you have a spinal fracture or some other problem, such as scoliosis (curvature of the spine) or degenerating disks. Any kind of spinal fracture is a warning sign: if you've had one fracture, you're at

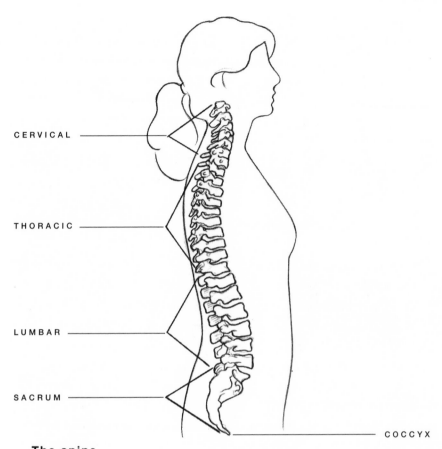

CERVICAL

THORACIC

LUMBAR

SACRUM

COCCYX

The spine

much greater risk to have another—so preventive measures are urgently needed. A diagnostic X ray can clarify the situation.

Talk to your doctor about bone density testing if you have any of the following symptoms:

- **Back pain:** This doesn't mean you have osteoporosis—back pain can result from many different causes, including muscle strain and nerve problems. Pain from osteoporotic fractures is usually felt in the middle or mid-upper back. Right after the fracture occurs, pain is often severe and sharply localized. But osteoporotic fractures also may produce milder and more diffuse discomfort.

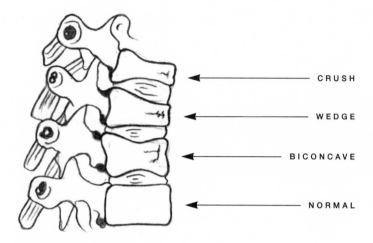

CRUSH

WEDGE

BICONCAVE

NORMAL

How the spine fractures

Crush fracture: The entire vertebra collapses. This kind of fracture often causes considerable back pain, as well as loss of height.

Wedge fracture: The front part of the vertebra is crushed but the back of the bone remains intact. Wedge fractures create the dowager's hump and bent-over posture characteristic of osteoporosis. They may also cause pain.

Biconcave fracture: The midsection of the vertebra collapses. This is often the first stage of a fracture that later becomes a wedge or crush. Biconcave fractures can cause pain.

- **Loss of height:** Women who suffer several fractures within a short period of time can lose height very quickly. When osteoporosis is severe and there are many fractures, total loss of height can amount to 5 to 8 inches. All women over age 35 should measure their height once a year, preferably in the morning (see box). Loss of more than an inch and a half of height can indicate vertebral fracture.

- **Stooped-over posture and dowager's hump:** These familiar and dreaded symptoms of osteoporosis are called **kyphosis.** The cause is usually wedge fractures in the spine. When the problem is mild, the woman may assume she simply has bad posture.

Clock your height

Your height actually varies through the day. You're at your tallest in the morning. During the day, gravity presses down on your spinal column, squeezing water out of the disks between your vertebras. As a result, you lose from a quarter to half an inch of height by the end of the day. Overnight, when you're lying in bed, the disks rehydrate. Since there's more variation in day-time activities than in sleep, your morning height is the most consistent.

◆ ◆ ◆

I went for a physical and the internist measured me. I was 5 feet 3½ inches. I used to be 5 feet 5½. I told the doctor, "I have to talk to you about osteoporosis." I notice a difference in my height. I can't get things out of the cupboard the way I used to. The cushions I got for my car and my ergonomic workstation no longer fit.

—KATIE

◆ ◆ ◆

No, you're not getting fat

Many times a woman with osteoporosis tells me, "I'm developing a tummy and I need to lose weight." But she hasn't gained weight and she's not fat. The problem is osteoporosis. Fractures have changed the shape of her spine, so the lower part curves toward the front of her body and pushes against her stomach and other internal organs. That's what's causing her protruding abdomen (and possibly indigestion and breathlessness too). Instead of dieting, she needs medication to address bone loss and exercises to strengthen her abdominal and postural muscles. These measures can make significant improvements.

There's no cure for a crushed vertebra, and no way to restore height or straighten a curved spine. But the back pain of osteoporosis can be treated—and further fractures may be prevented—by a combination of medication and exercise, as I'll explain in Chapters 8 and 9.

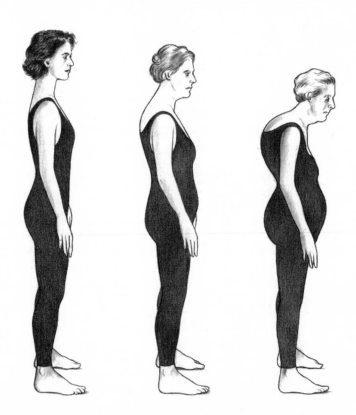

What osteoporosis looks like

These changes are not normal aging, but the effects of osteoporosis. As osteoporosis develops, a woman's height and posture change.

The wrist

Most osteoporotic fractures that occur in middle-aged women involve the wrist. Each year there are 250,000 wrist fractures in the United States. If you're over age 45, you have a 15 percent chance of fracturing your wrist eventually. Here's the most common scenario: A woman slips. She instinctively puts out her arm to break the fall—and she fractures her wrist.

Unlike fractures of the spine, wrist fractures are always too painful to go unnoticed. Diagnosis is confirmed by X ray. Most wrist fractures are treated by applying a cast that holds the bones in place until they heal. If the damage is more severe, the woman may need surgery to pin the bone. After the cast is removed, she may receive physical therapy to restore strength and flexibility.

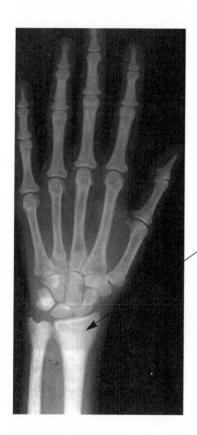

Wrist fracture

The arrow points to the site where most wrist fractures occur—at the end of the radius bone. This type of fracture is called Colles' fracture after Dr. Abraham Colles, who first described it over 170 years ago.

About half of women who suffer a wrist fracture recover completely after about two months of treatment and rehabilitation. But the remaining half experience lingering symptoms, including pain and weakness in the wrist and decreased range of motion. If the bones are pushed out of place, or if they don't heal perfectly, fractures also may leave the wrist permanently deformed or enlarged.

Like spinal fractures, a broken wrist is a valuable warning sign of bone loss. Women who've had a wrist fracture have twice the normal risk of vertebral and hip fractures. So preventive measures are urgently important.

The hip

Hip fractures are the most devastating consequence of osteoporosis, creating in many victims a downward spiral of complications from surgery and immobility. The older a woman is, the worse the consequences are likely to be.

I want to emphasize that having a hip fracture does *not* mean you're doomed to frailty and dependence! Medications, exercise, and good nutrition make an enormous difference. Some women not only recover their previous level of functioning but actually go on to become stronger and fitter.

◆ ◆ ◆

It was shortly after Christmas nine years ago. I was playing cribbage and the phone rang. I answered the call, then came running back—and slipped on the linoleum and broke my hip. My hip healed perfectly. A year and a half later, I went skiing and broke my leg on the same side, just below my knee. The doctor put me back together again.

Last winter I was disgusted to learn I had osteoporosis. How can you tell you have osteoporosis when you don't feel anything? I do a lot of exercising and strength training. I take Fosamax and supplements with calcium and vitamin D. I'm more cautious now. I'll accept assistance taking down the storm windows. I don't go downhill skiing anymore, just cross-country. But on the whole, I feel great.

—NANCY, AGE 80

◆ ◆ ◆

New treatments for broken bones

On the horizon are exciting new fracture treatments that could greatly speed the recovery process. At the moment, though, they're still under investigation.

- Synthetic bone cements have potential for treating fractured arm and leg bones and collapsed vertebras. The cement is injected into the broken bones, and new bone forms around it. Though this can't cure fractures—and the cements are difficult to work with—they may reduce pain, improve function, and prevent deformity.
- Ultrasound waves and electrical currents appear to stimulate repair of long bones—the bones in the legs and arms—after fracture. Patients use a small device in their own homes for twenty minutes a day. These techniques seem to be effective when the broken segments of bone don't join together well.
- Drug implants have been tried experimentally for treatment of broken long bones. A stimulating substance is implanted in a sponge-like material that is placed in the broken bone near the fracture. The implant appears to encourage bone growth and repair.

I've already explained how middle-aged women break a wrist when they fall. But as we get older we fall differently. Typically, an older woman moves more slowly. Instead of pitching forward when she stumbles, she collapses and falls to the side. Her reflexes are slower, so her arm may not shoot out. Even if it does, she may not be strong enough to stop her descent. So she lands on her hip. That's why there are many more hip fractures in women in their mid-seventies and older.

Hip fractures are always obvious: there's considerable pain; weight bearing is impossible. Ninety percent of hip fractures occur as a result of a fall. In the remaining cases, the bone breaks without trauma, and the fracture itself causes the fall. Though most women know right away what's happened, the diagnosis must be confirmed by X ray to determine the nature of the break and the most appropriate treatment.

Almost all hip fractures are treated surgically. If the bone is strong enough, a repair is made with screws and pins. Otherwise, the entire hipbone may be replaced by an artificial hip. Most patients require about a week of hospitalization and at least two to three months of rehabilitation therapy after a hip fracture.

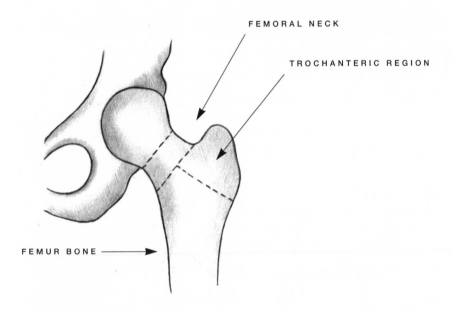

Hip fracture
The arrows point to the sites on the hip where fractures most frequently occur: the femoral neck and the trochanter.

Other fractures

Any bone can break because of osteoporosis, though fractures of the spine, wrist, and hip are the most common. If you fracture a bone after age 40, you might have osteopenia or osteoporosis. A bone density test can help you find out.

Can osteoporosis affect teeth?

By age 65, the average woman has lost six to eight permanent teeth, including her wisdom teeth. What does this have to do with osteoporosis? We've always assumed that older people lose teeth only because of cavities and gum disease. But we're discovering that bone loss is a factor too. It makes sense. When bone in the jaw becomes less dense, teeth aren't held as securely. So they may loosen and fall out. New research suggests that postmenopausal women who are on hormone replacement therapy lose fewer teeth as they age.

THE EMOTIONAL TOLL OF OSTEOPOROSIS

The pain and physical disabilities of osteoporosis are bad enough. But the emotional effects can be even worse. Ann says:

I was 44 years old. I'd just found out I was in menopause, and I wasn't prepared for it. When I got the news that I had osteopenia, I really freaked out. I felt fragile and scared. How many years would it take before I had osteoporosis?

Once I got the diagnosis, it seemed that osteoporosis was everywhere I turned. I ran into a woman in the grocery store, whom I hadn't seen for a year and a half, someone in her sixties who had always been full of life. Now she has osteoporosis. She looks so different. She's lost a lot of her height, and she's having a lot of pain.

A woman may be coping with unwelcome lifestyle changes: everyday activities, from cooking to sex, can become difficult or uncomfortable; her doctor may declare her favorite sports off-limits because she's at risk for fractures. Some women are embarrassed by their appearance; they may even avoid social situations rather than be seen by old friends. I wasn't surprised to read that when Canadian researchers asked women with osteoporosis to rate the importance of various problems associated with the disease, emotional issues were at the top. Indeed, fear of fractures—not pain—was number one. The women described anger and frustration, a sense of being overwhelmed, and a terrible fear of falling that limited their lives.

Anxiety and fearfulness are frequent problems for women with bone loss. Ann commented:

> *There's always an awareness there. I've never been a daredevil type, but now I'm a little bit more protective, a little bit more careful. People from my church play in a softball league. But you think, "If I got hit by a ball, will my leg break?" When you know you can't do something, you think, "Oh, that would have been fun."*

Sheila recalled:

> *I didn't tell people about my diagnosis. I just felt so old. I work in nursing homes, so I see the little bent-over old ladies. I thought, "Is this what I'm going to look like?"*

High on the list of emotional reactions reported by the Canadian women was anger. Sadly, most of the angry reactions I hear from women are directed against themselves. They wish they'd taken better care of their body when they were younger, or that they'd tested their bones earlier when they could have done more about prevention.

Depression and other emotional problems associated with osteoporosis often go undetected and untreated. That's a double tragedy. Negative emotions exacerbate the consequences of the disease, and can interfere with treatment. I hope that you won't hesitate to get professional help if you feel overwhelmed by osteoporosis.

The good news is that when women take charge of their condition—when they begin exercising, modify their diet, start medication—they feel in control again. Their physical symptoms improve, and their mood brightens as well. Liz—who was diagnosed with osteoporosis at age 42—has been taking Fosamax and supplements with calcium and vitamin D; she's also been strength-training. Two years later she reports:

I still have some pain, but there's a dramatic change compared to a year ago. I used to shuffle along, bent over. Now I walk with my back straighter; I feel more sure-footed. People who know me look at me and say, "Wow!" There's no question that my mood is better. I'm much happier. I feel better about everything.

Osteoporosis is a terrible disease. But I'm greatly encouraged by the long distance we've come in recent years—we're much more fortunate than our mothers and grandmothers. Whether we're trying to prevent the disease, or dealing with bone loss or fractures, there's so much we can do. It's never too early—or too late—to begin.

Osteoporosis Information Resources

The National Osteoporosis Foundation (NOF)
1232 22nd Street, N.W.
Washington, DC 20037-1292
800/223-9994
202/223-2226
http://www.nof.org

Osteoporosis and Related Bone Diseases Resources Center
National Institutes of Health
1232 22nd Street, N.W.
Washington, DC 20037-1292
800/624-BONE
202/223-0344
http://www.osteo.org

Foundation for Osteoporosis Research and Education (FORE)
300 27th Street, Suite 103
Oakland, CA 94612
888/266-3015
510/832-2663
http://www.fore.org

Men's Osteoporosis Online Support Group
http://pages.prodigy.net/jerryd3001/

Check Out
Your Bones

CHAPTER 4

Are You at Risk?

◆ ◆ ◆

A re you at risk for osteoporosis? If you're a woman, the answer is yes. *All* women are vulnerable to osteoporosis, and our vulnerability increases as we get older. But sex and age aren't the only risk factors for this disease. The full list is much longer. It includes some factors, such as your medical history, that are unavoidable. But others, like poor nutrition or smoking, can be addressed.

This chapter offers a simple questionnaire to help you assess your risk. I want to emphasize that adding up risk factors is *not* a substitute for bone density testing! Rather, my goal is to highlight areas where you can take charge of your bone health. The only way to find out if you actually have osteopenia or osteoporosis is to take one of the tests I'll describe in Chapter 5.

As you read this chapter, check the boxes that apply to you. Risk factors are cumulative, so each checked box indicates added risk. Pay particular attention to the shaded boxes—these are the risk factors that often can be modified.

DO YOU HAVE A FAMILY HISTORY OF OSTEOPOROSIS?

Check all the answers that apply to you:

My mother has (or had) osteoporosis. ☐

My father has (or had) osteoporosis. ☐

One or more siblings have (or had) osteoporosis. ☐

We now believe peak bone mass is determined 60 to 70 percent by genetic factors. So if either or both of your parents had osteoporosis and suffered fractures, you're at elevated risk too. And consider yourself warned if your older sister is diagnosed with osteoporosis.

The risk is even higher if your relative developed the problem relatively early in life. For instance, if your mother fractured her hip when she was 80 or older, you have double the average risk. But if she fractured her hip in her sixties or seventies, your risk is three times higher than usual.

Did your parents have osteoporosis?

Bone density testing wasn't available to the public until recently. In the past, doctors diagnosed osteoporosis only after a bone was broken—and sometimes not even then. Many women belatedly realize, from thinking back or looking at old photographs, that their parents probably had osteoporosis.

Here are some of the signs:

- Fracture of the hip, wrist, or pelvis
- Loss of height of more than an inch and a half
- Dowager's hump or hunched-over posture
- Chronic pain in the back

We don't know all the specific mechanisms involved in genetic risk for osteoporosis. Two likely factors are estrogen production and vitamin D metabolism. Your weight and body type—which are largely inherited, but also partly shaped by family lifestyle—are significant too.

HAVE YOU FRACTURED A BONE?

I broke a bone when I was 40 or older.   ☐

Studies consistently find that women who suffer fractures after age 40 either have osteoporosis or are at elevated risk of developing it. This is true regardless of which bone was broken, and even if the fracture was related to a trauma.

I have symptoms of spinal fracture.   ☐

Many women have spine fractures but don't realize it. These symptoms could indicate osteoporotic fractures in your spine: loss of height of more than an inch and a half, a dowager's hump, chronic pain in the middle or upper back.

WHAT IS YOUR RACIAL HERITAGE?

I'm Caucasian.   ☐

I'm Asian.   ☐

The lighter your skin, the greater your risk for osteoporosis. Here are the percentages of women over 50 of different races who have osteoporosis:

Caucasians and Asians	30 percent
Hispanics	16 percent
Blacks	10 percent

Scientists don't yet know all the reasons that black women enjoy this protection. Weight is one possibility—black women tend to be heavier, and they have more muscle as well as bone. But some studies find a persistent advantage, even when weight is taken into account.

I want to emphasize that black women are *not* immune to the problem. Like men, they simply develop it later. Among women age 90 and up, racial differences are very small. So prevention is important for everyone.

WHAT IS YOUR MENSTRUAL HISTORY?

Because estrogen is so important in bone formation, your lifetime exposure to estrogen is a good predictor of your bone mass: the higher your estrogen exposure, the more likely you are to have strong bones. The simplest way to approximate your estrogen exposure is to review your menstrual history.

I began to menstruate at age 15 or older.   ☐

Women who reach menarche (the beginning of menstruation) relatively late—age 15 and up—are at higher risk for osteoporosis.

Note: For mothers of teenage girls

By age 14, your daughter should be showing signs of puberty: budding breasts, hair under her arms, and menstruation. If these changes haven't appeared by the time she turns 15, discuss the situation with her doctor. There could be a medical problem that needs to be addressed. But some healthy girls simply develop unusually late.

I've experienced menstrual interruptions or irregularities.   ☐

Some women have menstrual irregularities that aren't caused by pregnancy, nursing, or impending menopause: their periods come infrequently or stop altogether. I'm not talking about an occasional delayed or missed period, but about a long-term or recurring pattern.

Menstrual interruptions or irregularities indicate lower estrogen exposure, which means elevated risk for bone loss. *A young woman who doesn't have menstrual periods can lose as much bone as a postmenopausal woman.*

Take menstrual abnormalities seriously. If hormonal issues are addressed, bone can be regained. Sometimes the problem is solved by nutritional changes and a slight weight gain. Medication, including birth control pills, may be used too.

Check all the relevant boxes:

I'm in menopause.   ☐

I reached menopause before age 45.   ☐

I entered menopause prematurely, when my ovaries
were removed.   ☐

All women are at increased risk of bone loss after menopause—but the risk is even higher for those who go through the change of life early (i.e., younger than age 45). That's because the earlier a woman stops menstruating, the less lifetime estrogen exposure she has. Even after menopause, the ovaries continue to manufacture some estrogen. So the risk of osteoporosis is slightly higher for a woman whose ovaries were removed. Hormone replacement therapy can compensate somewhat, but not fully.

WHAT IS YOUR BODY TYPE?

I'm tall and slender.   ☐

If Barbie ever grows older, she'll be at high risk for osteoporosis. Slender women generally have less bone mass than normal or heavy women, so they're particularly vulnerable to fractures—especially if they're also tall. The longer the bones, the easier it is for them to break. And of course, a tall woman has farther to fall.

Women who are tall and slender are at additional risk if they're underweight. Because we hear so many warnings about the dangers of excess weight, we sometimes forget that extreme thinness is unhealthy too—the problems include osteoporosis, and also elevated risk for cancer and infertility.

Being underweight works to the disadvantage of your bones in three ways:

- Very thin women tend to have lower-than-normal estrogen levels.
- Less force is applied to the bones—and mechanical force helps bones grow.
- Lower caloric intake means that a woman is less likely to get the nutrients she needs.

How can you tell if your weight puts you at risk? Measure your height, weigh yourself—and then look at the table to determine your body mass index (BMI). If your BMI is under 19, you're underweight. A BMI between 19 and 25 is healthy. If your BMI is over 26, your osteoporosis risk is actually lower than average.

My body mass index is under 19.   ■

WHAT IS YOUR DIETING HISTORY?

I've been a yo-yo dieter.   ☐

Yo-yo dieting—frequent cycles of losing and then regaining 15 or more pounds—puts you at increased risk for osteoporosis. That's because most people lose bone (and muscle) along with fat when they lose weight. We suspect that rapid weight loss is particularly detrimental to muscle and bone, because it triggers release of parathyroid hormone, which stimulates the bone-dissolving activity of the osteoclasts.

The best ways to counter these effects when you're dieting are to lose weight slowly (no more than a pound or two per week) and to do aerobic exercise and strength training to protect your muscles and bone mass.

I've suffered from an eating disorder.   ☐

Eating disorders—including both anorexia and bulimia—are very common in young women, especially athletes. Up to 30 percent of college varsity

BODY MASS INDEX (FOR WOMEN AND MEN)

1. Read down the first column to locate your height.
2. Read across that row and locate your weight.
3. Read the heading at the top of the column—that's your BMI range

HEIGHT (inches)	UNDERWEIGHT BMI under 19 (under this weight in pounds)	HEALTHY WEIGHT BMI 19 to 25 (within this range in pounds)	OVERWEIGHT BMI 26 or over (over this weight in pounds)
58	91	91–123	123
59	94	94–127	127
60	97	97–132	132
61	100	100–136	136
62	104	104–141	141
63	107	107–146	146
64	110	110–150	150
65	114	114–155	155
66	118	118–160	160
67	121	121–165	165
68	125	125–170	170
69	128	128–175	175
70	132	132–180	180
71	136	136–185	185
72	140	140–190	190

athletes experience some form of eating disorder, and the figure is even higher for elite competitors. Anorexic women lose their menstrual cycle (along with the bone benefits of estrogen); they're also underweight and they consume very little calcium. Bulimics may not be underweight and may continue menstruating, but their purging leads to calcium insufficiencies.

The effects of an eating disorder can be long-lasting, because the problem

An unexpected advantage

Women know that obesity carries many adverse health effects—including higher risk for cardiovascular disease, diabetes, breast and other forms of cancer, arthritis and joint problems. So they're often astonished to learn that excess weight is actually an advantage for bones.

One reason is mechanical: the heavier a woman is, the more stress she places on her bones with every step—and the more she stimulates them to develop. Over the years her bones adapt to the extra weight by becoming denser. Another factor is hormonal: fat cells produce a weak form of estrogen. This is a mixed blessing. While it benefits bone, extra estrogen increases the risk of breast and other cancers.

If a woman is at a healthy weight, experts do *not* recommend that she try to gain. Any advantage to her bones would be overshadowed by the disadvantages to other important areas of health. It's also important to note that overweight women are not immune to osteoporosis—they're simply at lower risk.

typically occurs during the teens and early twenties—years when young women normally are gaining bone. Women who suffer from an eating disorder may reach a lower than normal peak bone mass, reducing their margin of safety for later life.

DOES YOUR MEDICAL HISTORY PUT YOU AT RISK?

Medical problems—and the medications used to treat them—can affect bones. Below are some of the most common medical conditions that increase risk for osteoporosis. But this list is far from complete. If you have any kind of chronic medical condition, ask your doctor if it might affect your bones.

ABOUT THE RESEARCH

The athletic triad: amenorrhea, eating disorders, and bone loss

Women's participation in competitive sports increased dramatically in the 1970s and 1980s. I was a marathoner back then, and I knew that many of my fellow women runners were amenorrheic—that is, they'd stopped menstruating. This wasn't generally considered a problem at the time; indeed, many of the women regarded it as a convenience. Then in 1984 I read a disturbing finding from the University of California at San Francisco: Young athletic women who were amenorrheic had 20 to 30 percent lower bone density in their spine than athletes who menstruated.

My Tufts colleagues and I decided to investigate this finding further. We recruited twenty-eight women runners in their twenties and thirties. All ran at least 25 miles a week and were of normal weight. But eleven of the women hadn't menstruated for at least a year, while the rest had normal cycles. Bone density was significantly lower in the nonmenstruating women. These women also had 70 percent lower blood levels of estradiol, the most potent form of estrogen. Although none had an abnormally low BMI, they reported eating 500 calories less per day than the women who hadn't stopped menstruating. We noticed that many had disordered patterns of eating—for instance, some ate only one meal per day, or consumed many foods in unusually tiny portions, such as a teaspoon of cottage cheese or three almonds.

We published our findings in the *American Journal of Clinical Nutrition* in 1985. This was the first study to suggest a link between amenorrhea, disordered eating, and low bone density. Others have confirmed this pattern, which is now called the athletic triad. Ironically, it affects women who appear to be in superb physical condition, including dancers as well as athletes.

In another study, we looked at ninety-six elite women athletes—invited runners in the Boston Marathon. Though these were apparently healthy women in their twenties, thirties, and forties, 19 percent of them weren't menstruating. This time our focus was on stress fractures, a common injury among competitive runners. Thirty-six percent of the menstruating women had experienced one or more stress fractures. But the number was an alarming 72 percent for those who weren't menstruating—clear evidence that their bones were already compromised.

I suffer from rheumatoid arthritis.   □

Rheumatoid arthritis is an autoimmune disease. In other words, all the defense mechanisms of the immune system—which normally protect a person from disease—instead are directed against the woman's own body. One of the effects is extra osteoclast activity, with resulting loss of bone. The problem is exacerbated by the medications used to treat the disease. People with rheumatoid arthritis can lose bone rapidly.

Interestingly, women with osteoarthritis generally have a *reduced* risk of osteoporosis. The explanation could be that many people with osteoarthritis are overweight, which lowers their risk of osteoporosis. But there could be an as yet unknown genetic factor at work.

I have a thyroid disorder.   □

Individuals who suffer from hyperthyroidism, an overly active thyroid gland, are at higher risk for osteoporosis. Their excess thyroxin stimulates the bone-dissolving activity of the osteoclasts.

Ironically, a sluggish thyroid (hypothyroidism) is also a risk factor. In this case, the risk comes not from the disease itself but from the medications used to correct it. Until the dosage is properly adjusted, an individual may temporarily get too much.

I have a disorder of the parathyroid.   ☐

The parathyroid glands—four tiny glands in the neck—secrete parathyroid hormone (PTH), which plays an important role in bone remodeling. When too much PTH is secreted, osteoclast activity increases significantly, causing loss of bone.

I have Type 1 diabetes that is poorly controlled.   ☐

Adult-onset diabetes is not associated with osteoporosis. The relationship between Type 1 (childhood) diabetes and bone loss is not yet fully clear. Diabetics who are able to keep their condition under control don't seem to have elevated risk. But "brittle diabetics"—those who experience difficulty regulating their blood sugar—are more likely to develop osteoporosis.

I'm lactose-intolerant.   ☐

Some individuals experience bloating, cramps, or diarrhea if they consume dairy foods. That's because their bodies don't produce sufficient lactase, the enzyme needed to metabolize lactose, the sugar in milk and other dairy products. Since they can't tolerate these foods, they consume less of them—and their bones suffer as a result. Lactose intolerance is more common in black women, Asians, and Hispanics. That's one reason black women and Hispanics get osteoporosis, despite their genetic tendency to have strong bones. I'll discuss strategies for dealing with lactose intolerance in Chapter 7.

I suffer from a chronic digestive disorder.   ☐

Digestive problems—such as a food allergy, colitis, or Crohn's disease—make it harder for the body to absorb calcium. That means greater risk for osteoporosis.

DO YOU TAKE ANY MEDICATIONS THAT AFFECT YOUR BONES?

Even if a disease doesn't affect bone health, the medications used to treat it may have an impact. Below are some of the most common medications that weaken bones. If you take any other medication regularly, ask your doctor about its effects on bone.

I take a steroid.   ☐

Steroids (e.g., prednisone, cortisone) treat many conditions, including asthma, rheumatoid arthritis, ulcers, colitis, lupus, glaucoma, and HIV infection. They have a combination of effects that lead to bone loss: decreased absorption of calcium, increased urinary excretion of calcium, and also inhibited bone formation by the osteoblasts.

I take thyroid hormone.   ☐

Thyroid hormone, which is taken for hypothyroidism, increases bone breakdown unless the dose is properly calibrated.

I take medication for seizures.   ☐

Anticonvulsants are used to treat epilepsy and other seizure disorders. Some antiseizure medications can reduce bone density by interfering with calcium absorption.

I take a diuretic other than thiazide.   ☐

Diuretics are used to treat heart disease and high blood pressure. They increase urinary output, which also increases excretion of calcium. Thiazide is an exception: this diuretic preserves calcium. If you're using a blood pressure medication and have reason to be concerned about your bones, ask your doctor about switching to thiazide. Unfortunately, it's not potent enough for all medical conditions treated with diuretics.

I take a gonadotrophin-releasing hormone agonist. □

Fibroid tumors, endometriosis, and prostate cancer (in men) are treated with gonadotrophin-releasing hormone agonists, such as Lupron, which have an adverse effect on bone.

I use an antacid that contains aluminum. □

Antacids—which are available over the counter, as well as by prescription—treat heartburn, ulcers, and other ailments that cause indigestion. Some of these remedies contain aluminum, which interferes with calcium absorption if taken in excessive amounts.

When medicine is bad for your bones

Medications can be lifesaving. However, a drug that's helpful for one system of your body may cause adverse effects elsewhere. To find out, talk to your doctor and check the package insert. *If you discover a potential problem, don't stop taking the medication.* But ask your doctor these questions:

- Are there any alternatives to this medication?
- Can the dose be reduced?
- Can I drop or reduce the medication if my symptoms change?
- What can I do to counter the side effects on my bones?
- Should I be monitoring my bone density while I'm on this treatment?

DOES YOUR LIFESTYLE AFFECT YOUR BONES?

Physical exercise and good nutrition are critical for bone development—and for maintaining bone density as we grow older. Later in the book I'll give you information on bone-boosting activities, foods, and supplements.

Most days I'm sedentary, and spend less than thirty minutes at
moderate-to-vigorous physical activity.   ☐

The less active you are, the greater your risk for osteoporosis and fractures. Women who engage in any kind of regular exercise have stronger
bones; they also have better balance and coordination, which reduces their
risk of falling.

My daily diet typically does not include four servings of calcium-
rich foods.   ☐

There's a strong relationship between lifetime calcium intake and bone
density. Individuals who consume less than 600 milligrams of calcium per
day—approximately the amount in two glasses of milk—are at especially
high risk for osteoporosis.

I'm exposed to the sun for less than ten minutes per day, and don't
get vitamin D from supplements or fortified foods.   ☐

Vitamin D is essential for calcium metabolism, so low levels put you at
risk for osteoporosis. We get vitamin D from sun exposure, from diet (the
best sources are fortified milk and cereal), or from supplements. The sun
triggers cells in our skin to manufacture the vitamin. But in the wintertime,
sun exposure isn't sufficient. And as we get older, the body's ability to make
vitamin D is diminished. At those times, it becomes very important to get
enough via food or supplements.

Most days I don't eat five or more servings of fruits
and vegetables.   ☐

Women who consume plenty of fruits and vegetables have higher bone
density. Especially helpful for bone health are citrus fruits, which contain vitamin C, and green leafy vegetables, which provide vitamin K.

I consume more than seven alcoholic drinks
per week, on average.   ☐

Drinking more than seven alcoholic beverages per week is associated with increased risk of low bone density and fractures. Alcohol creates three different kinds of problems for bone:

- Alcohol decreases the bone-building activity of osteoblasts.
- High alcohol intake is associated with poor nutrition.
- Excess alcohol consumption has an adverse effect on balance, increasing the risk of falls and fractures.

I drink more than four cups of caffeinated coffee per day
(or get an equivalent amount from other sources).   ☐

Caffeine consumption over about 400 milligrams per day—the equivalent of four cups of coffee—doubles the risk of hip fracture. Caffeine has a diuretic effect, which increases excretion of calcium in the urine. Another concern is that caffeinated beverages may replace liquids that contain calcium.

Though coffee—with about 100 milligrams per cup—is the major source of caffeine for most Americans, it's not the only one. Tea has about 40 milligrams of caffeine per cup. Many people don't realize that soda often contains as much caffeine as tea (and nearly as much as coffee in some cases).

I'm a current or former smoker.   ☐

Smoking is one of the major risk factors for osteoporosis. Women with a smoking history have significantly lower bone density and are much more likely to suffer fractures than those who never lit up. That's because smoking decreases estrogen levels. Women who smoke tend to go through menopause earlier. If you've kicked the habit, congratulations! Your risk is considerably lower, though it remains higher than that of someone who never smoked.

YOUR RISK PROFILE

Osteoporosis risk is cumulative. Remember, you start at elevated risk just because you're a woman. Go back and review the clear boxes you checked—risk factors like your family and medical history, which are unavoidable. Now look at the shaded boxes. These represent risk factors you may be able to address. *The more unavoidable risk factors you have, the more important it is to minimize the risks you can control.*

I know from personal experience that it's alarming to realize you have osteoporosis risk factors you haven't thought about before. Even though I've been interested in bone since I was a child, and have worked professionally in this area for more than a decade, writing this chapter was an eye-opener for me. I eat well and get plenty of exercise, but other risk factors continue to operate. I realized once again that I'm not immune to osteoporosis.

Reviewing my risk profile gave me renewed motivation—and I hope it has a similar effect on you. No matter what your age or other risk factors, there is so much you can do to protect your bones and prevent osteoporosis.

Put Your Bones
to the Test

◆ ◆ ◆

A generation ago, the only practical way to find out if you were losing bone mass was to break a bone. Now you can take a simple fifteen-minute test and get a precise measure of your bone density. You can learn if your bones are dangerously weak without suffering a fracture, while there's still time for preventive measures.

Exciting as this advance is, I'm not suggesting that every woman rush out and have a bone density test right now. This chapter will help you decide when you need to be tested. I'll also describe the available procedures so you know what the options are and what to expect.

DO I NEED A BONE DENSITY TEST?

I hear this question often from concerned women. The answer depends on your age, your risk factors, and whether you're being treated for bone loss. We don't yet have a single set of guidelines, though there's considerable agreement among groups that have issued recommendations, including the National Osteoporosis Foundation, the American College of Obstetrics and Gynecology, and the American Association of Clinical Endocrinologists. The advice below is based on these guidelines. However, I believe that testing can benefit other women as well.

If you're about to start treatment for bone loss

A preliminary bone density test is standard practice before treatment starts. First, the test could help determine if you need medication. In addition, the test provides a baseline that allows you and your doctor to monitor the effectiveness of treatment.

If you have symptoms that suggest osteoporosis

Regardless of your age, ask your doctor about testing if you have symptoms that might indicate bone loss:

- You've had a fracture that suggests low bone density, because it was not related to a severe trauma.
- You've lost more than an inch and a half of height, or have developed curvature of the spine.
- You have acute or chronic pain in the middle to upper back.

Ironically, testing is often *not* recommended for an individual whose osteoporosis is readily diagnosed from age and severe symptoms—for instance, a woman in her nineties who has a history of fractures in her spine and has just broken her hip. The reason: Her doctor already knows that she needs treatment for osteoporosis, so test results wouldn't affect her care.

If you have significant risk factors

Some guidelines suggest testing for women in their twenties, thirties, or early forties if they have special risk factors:

- You've had your ovaries removed.
- You have a history of prolonged or chronic menstrual irregularities caused by a medical problem or an eating disorder.
- You have a medical condition that causes bone loss.
- You take a medication that harms bones, or are about to start such a medication.

What difference does a diagnosis make?

Most testing guidelines suggest that you have a bone density test only if the results will affect your course of action—for example, if you're taking the test to decide about medication or lifestyle changes. Though I see the logic of that position, I think it overlooks the motivational value of testing.

Some women tell me, "No matter what, I'm not going to stop smoking." Or, "I refuse to take medication." Often these same women reconsider when they face the reality of osteopenia or osteoporosis. Others tell me, "I'll start exercising when I'm not so busy." Then, after they review their test results, they suddenly find time for workouts.

You don't need a bone density test to know that you should be exercising and eating right to protect your bones. Nevertheless, I recommend testing even for women who think the results won't make a difference. Research shows that information often is a powerful motivator.

Getting tested now gives you precious extra time to protect your bones. If you have low bone density this early in your life, you might want to talk to your doctor about medication as well as nutrition and exercise.

If you're in perimenopause

Though most guidelines don't recommend testing at this time, I think it provides valuable information. As you approach menopause, bone loss accelerates. A baseline test will help you decide about hormone replacement and other protective measures during these critical years.

If you've gone through menopause

Guidelines generally recommend bone density testing for women over age 60 or 65, and for younger postmenopausal women who have one or more

What is perimenopause?

Perimenopause is the transition stage leading to menopause. It refers to the changes that most women notice in their forties, as hormone levels begin to fluctuate. Menstruation hasn't yet stopped, but periods become heavier or lighter, and the cycle is longer or shorter than normal. Some women experience occasional hot flashes, vaginal dryness, and other symptoms of menopause.

additional risk factors. But *all* women are at greatly increased risk for osteoporosis after menopause. Therefore, I urge you to consider testing if you're in menopause and haven't already been tested.

Bone density testing is particularly helpful if you're deciding about hormone replacement therapy (HRT). Also, if you've been on HRT and are thinking of stopping, you should know the condition of your bones.

Is it time for your first bone density test?

The answer is yes if:

- You have symptoms that suggest osteoporosis, such as fractures or loss of height.
- You need information to decide about beginning—or stopping— HRT or other treatment for your bones.
- You have significant risk factors other than being a woman.
- You're in menopause.

BONE-TESTING OPTIONS

Bone density is the best single predictor of future fractures. Density accounts for about 80 percent of the strength of your bones. Several different tests are used to measure bone density, which is also referred to as bone-mineral density or BMD. All these tests are safe, painless, quick (no more than ten to twenty minutes), and precise.

Depending on the kind of test you take, as well as your medical history, different bones will be measured. Though density scores of bones in different parts of the skeleton are usually closely correlated, some of your bones may be stronger than others. Differences could reflect your lifestyle—for instance, if you're a longtime racket sport player, the bones in your racket arm will be denser than average for your body. Or they could reflect genetic tendencies, just as the shape of your body does.

Dual X-ray absorptiometry (DXA)

The current test of choice is dual X-ray absorptiometry (called DXA or DEXA for dual energy X-ray absorptiometry). DXA is widely available and relatively inexpensive ($150 to $200); it can measure bone density in the hip, the spine, and the forearm. The hip and spine measurements are the ones usually done. They're particularly significant because that's where fractures have the most serious consequences. The greater your risk for osteoporosis, the more important this information is for you.

A smaller version of the DXA machine can measure bone density in the forearm and the heel. While this isn't quite as good as measuring the hip and spine directly, the results are very closely correlated. The test takes only two minutes, and the smaller machine can be used in community settings or doctors' offices, which makes it more convenient for many women.

Ultrasound densitometry

Another commonly available testing option is ultrasound. This technique uses a device no bigger than a suitcase; a test costs only $30 to $100 and in-

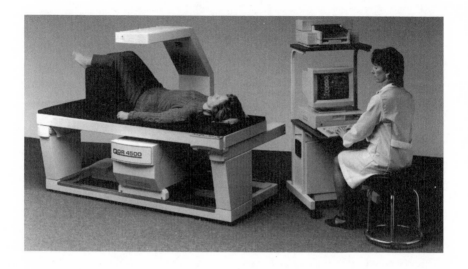

Dual x-ray absorptiometry (DXA)

You lie on a scanning table. When your spine is measured, as shown here, your legs are positioned on a firm pad to help flatten out your spine. For measurement of your hipbone, your legs lie flat on the table. During the test, the scanner moves back and forth over your body.

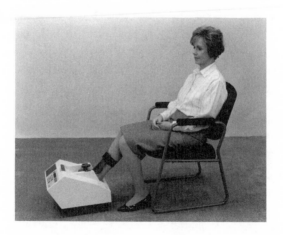

Ultrasound densitometry

You're seated with your foot in the device. It sends sound waves through your foot, and measures what is absorbed by the bone and other tissues in your heel. Some devices place your foot in a water bath to help conduct the sound waves.

volves no radiation. Thanks to ultrasound technology, someday women may be able to test their bones at the corner drugstore. Ultrasound testing is already available in many doctors' offices around the country.

Unfortunately, ultrasound can't check bone density in the spine and hip. The site most commonly measured is the heel; other bones in the lower leg and hand can be checked too. The results reflect not only density but also properties of collagen in the bone. While this information is helpful because the results are strongly correlated with fracture risk, it's not a substitute for direct measurement of hip or spine bone density with DXA.

How the tests work

DXA uses a technique called **densitometry** or **X-ray absorptiometry;** the machine passes an X-ray beam through an area of bone. Ultrasound testing uses sound waves instead of X rays. Radiation (or sound waves) are absorbed by the bone—the denser the bone, the more it absorbs. The machine's detectors translate absorption information into a measure of bone density.

The "dual" in dual X-ray absorptiometry (DXA) refers to the use of two different X-ray beams, which enables the machine to distinguish between bone and the soft tissue (e.g., muscle, fat) covering it. That's why DXA can measure density of the hip and spine bones, even though they lie deep inside the body. Tests that use just a single beam can only measure bones that are just under the skin, such as the bones in the hand, wrist, and heel.

Other bone density tests

Other bone density tests are available, but used less frequently than DXA or ultrasound. Please note: This is an exploding field, and I expect to see many more options in the near future. Bone density testing should become even more convenient and informative, and even less expensive. That's great news for women.

Single X-ray absorptiometry (SXA)

Now that DXA is available, SXA—which can't check spine and hip bones—has been phased out. SXA measures bone density in the fingers, wrist, and heel. Those results correlate strongly with hip and spine density, so the test remains a good general indicator of bone health.

Radiographic absorptiometry (RA)

Radiographic absorptiometry (RA) is a special type of X ray. It measures bone density in the hand, which is closely correlated with hip and spine density. The chief advantage of RA is low cost. Also, nearly any X-ray machine can be adapted for RA. This makes it a valuable screening tool for women without easy access to DXA, such as those who live in remote rural areas.

Computerized axial tomography (CT or CAT scan)

CT scans are used mainly in research. But they can be helpful when other tests aren't available, or in special situations. DXA, SXA, X ray, and RA all produce a two-dimensional image of the bone. CT also uses an X-ray beam, but it can create a three-dimensional image. That can be important when a woman appears to be losing significantly more trabecular than cortical bone. In such a case, a CT scan would allow separate examination of the trabecular bone in the center of her spine.

HOW TO INTERPRET YOUR TEST RESULTS

The results of a bone density test can be a little confusing at first glance. But once you know how to interpret the numbers and graphs, you'll find the results very informative. Here's a guide to the terminology:

Bone-mineral density (BMD)

All of the tests measure the amount of mineral in a specific area of bone. The more mineral, the denser the bone. Mineral is measured in grams; area is measured in square centimeters—and BMD is described as grams per square centimeter, or g/cm^2.

T-score

The T-score compares your bone density with that of the average healthy young adult woman. T-scores are based on a statistical measure called the standard deviation, which reflects differences from the average score.

T-SCORE	STATISTICALLY SPEAKING	WHAT THAT MEANS	DIAGNOSIS
Higher than −1	Your bone mass is within 1 standard deviation of the average for healthy young adult women, or better.	Your bone mass and your risk of fractures are average or better. Eighty-five percent of healthy young adult women are in this range.	Adequate bone density
Between −1 and −2.5	Your bone mass is between 1 and 2.5 standard deviations lower than the average for healthy young adult women.	Your bone mass is lower than normal, and your fracture risk is approximately twice as high as average. The lowest 1 to 14 percent of healthy young adult women have bone density this low.	Osteopenia
Less than −2.5	Your bone mass is lower than the average for healthy young adult women by more than 2.5 standard deviations.	Your bone mass is very low—lower than 99 percent of healthy young adult women. Your risk for fractures is approximately three times higher than average.	Osteoporosis

Z-score

As we get older, we usually lose bone. So our T-scores normally drop. The Z-score presents our BMD in a different way—as a comparison with women our own age. A low Z-score is a warning that we're losing bone more rapidly than our peers, so we need to be monitored more closely.

Z-SCORE	STATISTICALLY SPEAKING	WHAT THAT MEANS
Higher than −1	Your bone mass is within 1 standard deviation of the average for women your age, or better.	Your bone mass is within or above the normal range for women your age.
Between −1 and −2.5	Your bone mass is between 1 and 2.5 standard deviations lower than the average for women your age.	Your bone mass is lower than average for your age. Compared to your peers, you're in the lowest 1 to 14 percent.
Less than −2.5	Your bone mass is lower by more than 2.5 standard deviations than the average for women your age.	Your bone mass is much lower than average—lower than 99 percent of women your age.

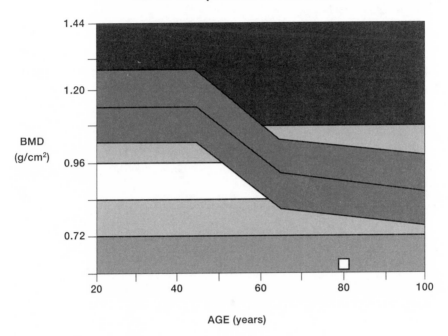

L2-L4 Comparison to Reference

Region	BMD g/cm²	Young-Adult %	T	Age-Matched %	Z
L2-L4	0.637	53	−4.7	70	−2.2

How to read BMD test results

Nina is an 80-year-old woman. Her doctor suggested DXA scans after she fractured her wrist. Here are the test results for her spine, and what they mean.

L2–4 are the second, third, and fourth bones of the lumbar spine (see diagram of the spine on page 35). These bones are used because they are the easiest part of the lumbar spine to measure consistently.

BMD (g/cm²) is bone mineral density, which is measured in grams per square centimeter.

The two zigzag parallel bands represent the usual range of bone density for women of different ages. The center line is the average; the bands show the range 1 standard deviation above and below. Bone density is stable from the twenties to mid-forties, dips sharply until the mid-sixties, then declines more slowly.

The shaded horizontal bands that run straight across the graph represent healthy bone, osteopenia, osteoporosis, and severe osteoporosis.

Nina's BMD is represented by the white square. Its position shows that she has severe osteoporosis, and that her bone density is much lower than average for a woman age 80.

Nina's T-score is −4.7, which indicates severe osteoporosis of the spine. Her spine has 53 percent of the bone density of a healthy young woman. This means she's lost almost half of the bone she had in her twenties and thirties.

Nina's Z-score is −2.2, which underscores the severity of her osteoporosis: even compared with other 80-year-olds, she has unusually low bone density—only 70 percent of the average for her age.

The DXA results for her hip also showed severe osteoporosis. Based on these and other findings, Nina's doctor prescribed calcium, vitamin D, and Fosamax. She will be tested again in a year to see if this treatment is effective.

◆   ◆   ◆

I had a DXA, and there was significant bone loss. My T-score for my hip was −3.78. The technician was very nice. He showed me the picture and said, "See those black spots? Those are holes in your hipbone."

—LAURA

◆   ◆   ◆

OTHER IMPORTANT TESTS

Bone density tests are the best way to determine if you have osteopenia or osteoporosis. But these tests can't tell you *why* you're losing bone or how fast it's happening. Nor can they evaluate suspected spine fractures or broken bones. So your doctor may suggest one or more additional tests. Here are some possibilities.

X ray

X rays are the most accurate way to detect and assess bone fractures. If you break your hip or wrist, or if you have symptoms of spinal fractures, your doctor probably will suggest a diagnostic X ray.

Bone turnover tests

Bone density changes so slowly that tests usually don't show results for at least a year. Doctors can check treatments more quickly via blood or urine tests that measure various by-products of remodeling. These tests can sometimes determine how rapidly the osteoclasts are breaking down bone, and how effectively the osteoblasts are restoring it.

Hormone tests

Blood tests can check levels of hormones important to bone, including:

Estradiol

This is the most potent form of estrogen. If you're under age 45 and experiencing menstrual irregularities, your doctor may check your estradiol and other estrogens. If levels are abnormally low, birth control pills might be suggested to boost your supply of estrogen, thereby protecting your bones.

Follicle-stimulating hormone (FSH)

FSH is a pituitary hormone that stimulates the ovaries, indirectly affecting estrogen supplies. As a woman approaches menopause, her FSH levels normally rise. Checking FSH helps your doctor determine if you're entering menopause. This narrows down possible causes of amenorrhea and other menstrual irregularities.

Thyroid and parathyroid

Problems with the thyroid and parathyroid glands can lead to bone loss. Thyroid or parathyroid hormone tests are the first diagnostic step when these issues are suspected.

Calcium metabolism tests

Abnormalities in blood calcium levels don't necessarily mean that you have osteoporosis, but they can help clarify your medical situation. For example, some parathyroid problems cause an increase in blood calcium.

THE PRACTICALITIES

I hope that bone density testing becomes a part of your routine health care, along with mammograms and Pap tests. You've already learned when to schedule your first test and what the options are. Here are answers to other common questions:

How often should I be tested?

Bones change slowly, so you don't need to check them very often. Indeed, the results could be misleading if you repeat a test too soon. Most of these tests are accurate to within 1 percent, which means that a change of less than 2 percent might simply reflect measurement errors. Though this is excellent accuracy for a medical test, the changes you might expect to see in your bones are small too. That's why very frequent testing is not advised.

After your first bone density test, I suggest testing every two or three years, except under these circumstances:

- If you're starting treatment for osteopenia or osteoporosis, have annual tests for the first three years to monitor effectiveness. Afterwards, testing every two or three years usually suffices. Your doctor may want more frequent tests if you're changing treatments or if you continue to have rapid bone loss. Less frequent tests might be suggested if you're younger and your bones have been stable.
- If you took your first bone density test before your mid-forties simply to obtain a baseline, and your bone density was normal or above normal, you don't need another test until you enter menopause—unless you develop a significant new risk factor for osteoporosis. After menopause, have tests every two years.

- If your bone density is well above average, and you have no major risk factors other than your age and the fact that you're a woman, tests can be done less frequently.

Where should I go for testing?

DXA and ultrasound are now available throughout the United States. Your doctor probably can refer you to a testing site in your area. Or you can find one yourself. Call the women's health department at the nearest teaching hospital and ask for a suggestion.

Once you've had a test, return to the same site for future measurements if possible. Though all testing methods are quite accurate, different machines are calibrated slightly differently. Since you're looking for small changes when you monitor your bones, it's best to stick with the same facility for subsequent tests.

Will my health insurance pay for testing?

The best way to find out is to ask your insurance company or health care provider. The answer depends not only on the terms of your coverage but also on your medical history. Bone density testing is likely to be covered by insurance if:

- You are postmenopausal and have risk factors, or you're 65 or older.
- You have vertebral abnormalities or have suffered a fracture that probably was caused by osteoporosis.
- You're at high risk for osteoporosis because of a medical condition or long-term treatment with steroids or other medications known to cause bone loss.
- You're about to start an FDA-approved treatment for osteoporosis.

If your medical insurance doesn't pay for bone density testing—but you feel it's important for your health—I encourage you to take the test, even if you have to cover the cost yourself. Preventing a fracture is worth a lot. Knowing your bone density can help you and your doctor decide what preventive measures or treatments you need.

Even if you're not covered now, you might be in the future. Medicare, HMOs, and private insurers are reassessing their policies, not only under pressure from worried women but also because testing and early diagnosis are cost-effective. Fractures are expensive too!

When to make the appointment

Your bone density changes with the seasons. These changes can actually be larger than what you'd expect from treatment, so it's important to have your bones retested at the same time of year (i.e., within a four-week period). Otherwise the comparison could simply reflect seasonal differences in sunlight exposure.

How to make your case

Insurers are more likely to cover testing for women under age 65 if they have risk factors for bone loss or if they're considering therapy. Talking to your doctor ahead of time can help you strengthen your case for reimbursement.

Before you discuss testing with your doctor, review the risk factors you checked in Chapter 4. For instance, if you're 45, you might not think to mention that you were hospitalized for an eating disorder at age 18 and stopped menstruating for two years. But this is relevant information. The more risk factors you have, the more likely it is that your insurance will pay for your test.

If you're perimenopausal or postmenopausal and under age 65, and you don't have other significant risk factors, you're a candidate for HRT. You might tell your doctor that you're concerned about your bones, and that a bone density test would help you decide about HRT or other therapy.

. . .

When our mothers were our age, they had no practical way to measure the density of their bones. Today, excellent tests are widely available. Very few diagnostic tests of comparable importance to our well-being are as easy and reliable as bone density tests. I urge you to discuss testing with your doctor. The information you obtain will make all the difference in preventing or treating osteoporosis.

Falling—
the Forgotten Factor

◆ ◆ ◆

O steoporosis makes bones vulnerable. But this vulnerability doesn't usually cause fractures all by itself. That's why it's critically important to prevent falls. About 90 percent of osteoporosis-related hip fractures—and more than 90 percent of wrist and pelvic fractures, and about half of spinal fractures—result from falls.

Most young people give little thought to falling, unless they engage in risky sports like skiing or in-line skating. But falling—and the fear of falling—become an ominous presence in many women's lives as they grow older. Indeed, falls are the leading cause of accidental death in people over age 65. However, you'll be encouraged to learn how much you can do to reduce your risk of falls.

We used to think that poor balance didn't become a problem until age 70 or so. But we now know it starts much earlier. This chapter has many tests that will help explore your balance. I think the results will fascinate and surprise you.

FALLING THROUGH LIFE

Y ou already know that we tend to lose bone as we get older. We also lose our ability to stay in balance. These combined changes dramatically increase the risk of falls and fractures.

Children, teens, and young adults generally have excellent balance. They rarely fall or suffer fractures from everyday activities. Balance begins to deteriorate in the mid-forties. Changes are subtle and happen slowly, so we may not be aware of them. But health statistics show a rise in fractures for women starting around age 45. This reflects loss of both bone and balance.

By the mid-sixties, changes in balance are obvious. Women feel less steady on their feet and they fall more frequently. Each year, about a third of women over age 65—and half of women age 80 and up—experience a fall.

Fear of falling becomes a significant problem. Many women—even those who haven't fallen—curtail their activities to avoid falls. This diminishes their quality of life, and also leads to inactivity, which causes further weakness and increases the risk of falls.

◆ ◆ ◆

I have osteoporosis. I'm 44, but doctors give me the kind of advice they probably give 80-year-old women: "You can take walks, but be careful not to fall." I can still hike, but no more jogging. I have three kids, and I'd always wanted to try downhill skiing and ice-skating when they were old enough. Now I can't. If I fall, I may wind up in a wheelchair.

—LAURA

◆ ◆ ◆

HOW GOOD IS YOUR BALANCE?

This question may already trouble you. Or perhaps you still take for granted your ability to move and remain upright. But even if you think your balance is excellent, it's helpful to try the tests below. You'll become more aware of your balancing ability and how it works, which will be useful as you read this chapter.

It's helpful to have a stopwatch or a clock with a second hand when you take the tests. For the more advanced tests, which are performed with your

How we know about falls

When you read the statistics in this chapter, you may wonder how scientists know about the frequency of falls. Most people fall at home; often they don't get hurt, so there's no need to tell a doctor.

The answer: Several comprehensive studies have carefully followed large groups of older men and women to find out how often they fall. One of the best was a 1989 project by John Campbell, M.D., in Dunedin, New Zealand—a town where nearly everyone is registered at a single health center. Dr. Campbell and his associates gained the cooperation of 92 percent of the town residents age 70 and up, a total of 761 people. Each participant agreed to fill out a form every time they fell. In addition, a nurse called everyone once a month to ask about falls; if an individual suffered from memory loss, a relative was called. The investigators also examined hospital records to check for injuries. Fall-prevention programs are based on this and other studies of falling.

eyes closed, you'll need a spotter—someone to stand nearby and steady you if necessary. The tests are fun, but they become quite challenging. Please be careful! It's very important to observe these cautions:

- Perform the tests in the order given, since they're arranged by degree of difficulty. *If you can't do one of the tests, do not attempt the rest—you could fall and hurt yourself.*
- Stand near a counter so you can catch yourself if necessary. Remember that you must have a spotter if you try the tests with your eyes closed.
- Wear sturdy, supportive shoes without heels, such as sneakers. Good shoes add to your stability.
- Practice once or twice before you take a test. But don't try the next test unless you can pass the one before.

If you're uncertain of your balance, take this preliminary test: Stand in front of the counter with your feet side by side and touching. Can you remain in that position for ten seconds, without using your hands for support? If not, your balance is extremely poor. *Do not attempt the other tests.*

Test 1: Tandem stand

Stand to the side of the counter, and put your hand on it for support. Position one foot directly in front of the other; the heel of the front foot should be just touching the toes of the foot in back. Try to distribute your body weight evenly on your two feet. Steady yourself and let go of the counter. Hold this position for ten seconds, without the aid of your hands. Your toes may wriggle slightly during the test, subtly redistributing your weight to maintain your balance. But your feet should not leave the floor.

If you can't complete this test, your balance is very poor. *Don't try the other tests.*

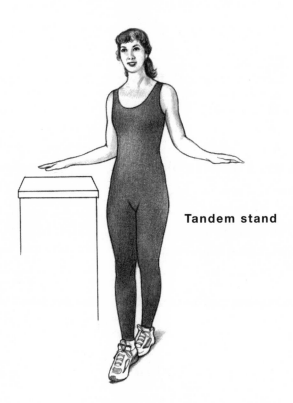

Tandem stand

Test 2: One-legged stand

Stand to the side of the counter with your feet together. Put your hand on the counter for support. Shift your weight to one foot. Bend the other knee to bring that foot up in back. When you're balanced on one leg, let go of the counter—but keep your hands poised so you can catch yourself if necessary. Hold this position for ten seconds.

Test 3: Tandem stand with eyes closed

This is the same as Test #1—except that your eyes will be closed. *Do not try this test unless you have someone to spot you.*

Stand to the side of the counter, and put your hand on it for support. Position one foot directly in front of the other; the heel of the front foot should be just touching the toes of the foot in back. Try to distribute your body weight evenly on your two feet. Close your eyes. Steady yourself and let go of the counter. Attempt to hold the position for ten seconds. You will be surprised at how much more difficult it is to balance when your eyes are closed!

Test 4: Tandem stand with eyes closed and head turning

This adds an additional challenge to Test 3. *Again, you will need a spotter.*

Stand to the side of the counter, and put your hand on it for support. Position one foot directly in front of the other; the heel of the front foot should be just touching the toes of the foot in back. Try to distribute your body weight evenly on your two feet. Close your eyes. Steady yourself and let go of the counter. Slowly turn your head to the right; then slowly turn it all the way to the left, and then return to face front. Take about ten seconds to complete the turns from right to left to center.

Test 5: One-legged stand with eyes closed

This is the same as Test 2, except your eyes are closed. *You must have a spotter.*

Stand to the side of the counter with your feet together. Put your hand on the counter for support. Shift your weight to one foot. Bend the other knee to bring that foot up in back. When you're balanced on one leg, close your eyes. Let go of the counter—but keep your hands poised so you can catch yourself if necessary. Try to hold this position for ten seconds. It's considerably harder than you might expect!

IF THE HIGHEST TEST YOU COULD PASS WAS:	YOUR BALANCE IS:
Test 5: One-legged stand with eyes closed	Excellent
Test 4: Tandem stand with eyes closed and head turning	Very good
Test 3: Tandem stand with eyes closed	Good
Test 2: One-legged stand	Fair
Test 1: Tandem stand	Poor
Unable to pass any tests	Very poor

There are no standardized performance scores for balance. But based on my experience with women ranging from active young adults to the frail elderly, I'd expect a fit, healthy woman under age 35 to score "excellent" with a little practice. If you're between 35 and 50, with no physical handicaps, you should rate "good." Older women might expect to have "fair" balance—though many active women in their fifties, sixties, and even seventies and eighties can do better. For a frail woman in her eighties or nineties, passing Test 1 is challenging.

Please don't be discouraged if your results were disappointing. Regardless of your age, you can improve your balance significantly. In Chapter 8, you'll learn how.

WHAT KEEPS US UPRIGHT?

As you know from the tests, good balance depends on your vision. Balance also requires fitness and agility, since we must constantly shift our weight to maintain equilibrium.

Balance and the senses

The brain receives information about our position from three different sensory systems. We can remain standing even if one or two of the systems aren't working perfectly. But we need all three for optimal balance.

Somatosensory system

Receptors on the skin and in the muscles and joints tell the brain where we are in our environment. Have you ever tried to walk when your foot has fallen asleep and is temporarily numb? Without information from nerves in your feet, it's very difficult to be steady.

How's your proprioception?

Proprioception is your sense of where you are in space. Here's a simple test to check this ability:

Sit in a comfortable chair that's more than an arm's length away from other objects. Close your eyes and put your left arm out to your side. Keeping your eyes closed, touch your left fingertip to your nose. Do the same with your right hand. If your fingertip landed in the wrong place, even after a few practice tries, mention this to your doctor at your next checkup.

Vision

If you attempted the tests with your eyes shut, you understand the enormous importance of vision for balance. Our eyes help our brain know where we are in space and whether we're upright. So cataracts, macular degeneration, or any other kind of impaired vision compromises our balance.

Vestibular system in the inner ear

Your inner ears are filled with fluid that plays a key role in balance. As your head moves, this fluid sloshes against receptors that signal the brain. The tests that involved turning your head demonstrated the importance of this system.

Do you have unsteady vision?

Ask yourself if you experience these minor problems more often than other people—or more often than your younger self:

- Do you trip when you're walking?
- Do you bump into obstacles, such as the corner of a coffee table?
- Do you stumble because you misjudge steps or sidewalk curbs?
- Do you accidentally knock over objects, such as a wineglass or a table lamp?
- Do you hit your head when you're getting out of a car?

"Yes" answers to any of these questions could reflect vision problems. Good vision isn't just a matter of being able to read letters on an eye chart; it has to do with depth perception and ability to see contrasts. Have your vision checked regularly, and make sure it's corrected as well as possible. This is especially important if you wear bifocals.

An ear for good balance

Here's a test of your vestibular system, which you can perform if you scored at least "good" on the balance test. The room should be quiet. Your eyes will be closed, so it's important to have a spotter. *Interrupt the test if you feel unsteady!*

Mark a spot on the floor and stand on it. Close your eyes and march in place for one minute. Try to remain on the spot as you march. When the minute is up, open your eyes and see if you've held your position. If you've drifted more than a foot to the left or right, you might have a vestibular problem. Mention the test to your doctor at your next checkup.

Balance and fitness

Have you ever lost your balance because you misjudged the bottom of a flight of stairs? Your somatosensory system felt your foot slip out from under you. Your eyes observed that your surroundings were moving too quickly. And your vestibular system sensed that you were no longer upright. Emergency!

In a flash, your brain went into action to keep you from falling. Sensory information was integrated rapidly, and commands were issued to your muscles. Without thinking, you staggered forward and flailed your arms, struggling to regain your balance. If your muscles were strong and flexible, and if your reaction time was quick, you avoided a fall. I hope so!

People who are fit and active have better balance and fewer falls. Three aspects of fitness are especially important:

Lower-body strength

If you're sitting in a sturdy kitchen or dining room chair, can you stand up without assistance from your hands? This simple test of lower-body strength is one of the best ways researchers have found to predict falls. If you can't pass, your risk of falling is two or three times higher than normal. Strength training can make significant improvements, even if you're frail.

Ankle strength and flexibility

Weak, inflexible ankle joints significantly increase your risk for falls. If your ankles can't bend easily, it's easier to lose your balance and harder to catch it again. Are your ankles up to the job? Take these two tests to find out. They require a ruler and a friend. If you need to improve, exercises in Chapter 8 will help.

Test 1: Stand facing a counter, with your feet shoulder-width apart. Put your hands on the counter to help you balance. Your friend should be at your feet with the ruler. Stand up on the balls of your feet. If your ankles are flexible, you should be able to raise your heels at least 2 inches off the ground.

Test 2: Stand with your back to a wall, your feet about 4 inches away. Your shoulders and buttocks should touch the wall. Try to lift your toes and the balls of your feel off the floor, so you're standing on your heels. If your ankles are strong and flexible, you'll be able to raise the balls of your feet at least 1½ inches off the floor. Note: Most people find this test much more difficult than the first one.

Rapid reaction time

Quick reflexes prevent falls. If you get off balance, your body doesn't have much time to react. You probably know if you react quickly, from everyday events such as trying to catch a dish that's just fallen off a counter.

Scientists use sophisticated computer programs to test reaction time. But here are two simple tests you can do at home. The first requires a stopwatch; if you don't have one, do the second test instead.

Test 1 (with a stopwatch): Start the watch, then stop it as close to five seconds as you can. Practice a few times, then take the test. Your reaction time is quick if you can consistently stop the clock between 4.9 and 5.1 seconds.

Test 2 (without a stopwatch): You'll need a friend and a crisp dollar bill. Stand facing your friend. Ask her to hold the bill by one of the short edges. Position your fingers on either side of the middle of the bill, an inch away. Then ask your friend to count, "One-two-three-drop," and drop the bill. If your reaction time is quick, you should be able to grab it after a couple of practice attempts. If you pass the test, try it without the "One-two-three" warning.

OTHER RISK FACTORS FOR FALLING

The risk of falling is affected by factors other than senses and fitness. Many of these risk factors are also associated with aging. But as you'll see, much can be done to address them.

Medical conditions

Physical problems can have adverse effects on balance. Because balance is not the primary symptom, you may not notice that it's affected. Here are some common examples:

Osteoporosis

Osteoporosis itself is a risk factor for poor balance. Fractures in the spine can cause bent-over posture. If the head—which is very heavy—is in front of the body rather than perched on top, the center of gravity shifts forward and balancing becomes more difficult.

Overweight and significant changes in weight

Overweight women are more likely to have balance problems because of the extra demand on their muscles—more strength is required to keep a heavier body in line. Weight changes, up or down, can also affect balance. Pregnant women sometimes feel unsteady as they gain weight. And women who have undergone mastectomy can feel unbalanced if they don't use a weighted prosthesis.

Arthritis

Any condition that limits mobility also impairs balance. People with arthritis are more vulnerable to trips and falls. Compounding the problem is their reduced strength and flexibility.

Neurological disorders

Balance may be impaired by conditions that affect the brain, the somatosensory system, or balance reflexes. Impaired balance is one consequence of Parkinson's disease and other neurological disorders.

Low blood pressure (hypotension)

Abnormally low blood pressure can cause dizziness or loss of balance. Normally the body adjusts blood pressure to changes in position. But some people experience a precipitous drop in blood pressure when they stand up or move after standing still for a few minutes. This condition, which is called **postural hypotension,** can cause dizziness.

Medications

Doctors may not consider balance when they prescribe medications for unrelated conditions, but drugs can have side effects that contribute to falls. Be aware of balance issues if you take any of the following:

- A drug that causes sleepiness, such as a sedative or narcotic painkiller
- Mood-altering medication, such as antidepressants or tranquilizers
- Medication for high blood pressure, including diuretics (these can cause low blood pressure)

Polypharmacy

Do you take many different prescription medications? That's called polypharmacy, and it's a warning flag to balance specialists. Many studies have found a strong association—which is only partially explained by illness—between taking more than four medications and falling.

Older people often are treated by several different doctors, and receive one or more prescriptions from each. Unless the physicians coordinate their efforts, the result can be unwanted side effects—including balance problems—from excessive medication or harmful drug interactions. If you're taking more than four prescription drugs, don't stop! But keep a master list and ask your primary doctor to review it from time to time, to see if you could cut back. Also, give a copy to each doctor who treats you.

Risky sports

Even world-class athletes—men and women in superb physical condition—are vulnerable to falls if they engage in challenging sports like ice-skating, gymnastics, or rock climbing. Falls are common in less obviously risky sports too. For instance, it's easy to slip if you're sprinting and stretching to return a fast tennis serve.

If you're a weekend athlete, be aware that you become more vulnerable to injuries—including falls—as you get older. Add balance and strength training to your weekday workouts, even if you're getting plenty of exercise on the weekend. If you aren't already active, it's important to get fit before you take up challenging sports.

Alcohol

Loss of balance is one of the most obvious effects of excess alcohol consumption—that's why people suspected of drunk driving are asked to walk a straight line. We use the same test in the lab to assess balance. Long-term alcohol abuse can damage the brain and affect balance even when a person is sober. The elderly and others who start with a balance deficit are particularly vulnerable to the effects of alcohol.

Footwear

One of the easiest ways to protect your bones is to change your shoes. Best for balance are sturdy, supportive shoes of canvas or leather that are held snug to the foot with laces or Velcro. Heels should be low. Soles should be flexible and not so thick that you can't feel the ground.

About 50 to 60 percent of falls happen because the person trips—and shoes are often a contributing factor. A study by researchers in Birmingham, England, implicated improper footwear in nearly 45 percent of falls in older adults. That may sound like a lot, but it's consistent with what I've seen in my work with elderly women.

Many people (especially women) wear shoes like these, which increase the risk of falls:

- Platform shoes, clogs: Thick soles interfere with proprioception—your ability to feel the ground you're walking on.
- Sneakers with thick treads: Though designed to give you good traction outdoors, thick treads become a hazard indoors, especially when walking on a rug.
- High heels: Height makes you tippier. Also, the heels reduce the surface area on which your weight must balance.
- Mules and other open-back shoes: You're less stable if your heels are allowed to slide.
- Loose boots: These give little or no support.
- Old footwear: After years of use, shoes become less sturdy, and soles become slippery.

Common household hazards

Nearly half of all falls take place in the home—and approximately 85 percent of those are caused by environmental hazards. When you opened a book on osteoporosis, you probably didn't expect to be warned about dim lightbulbs, throw rugs, and floor polish. But anything that contributes to falling is a threat to your bones. You can greatly reduce the odds of a fracture by giving your home a safety checkup, and correcting any problems you find. This is helpful for any household, but it's especially important for residences where an older person lives or visits.

Floors
- Avoid polishes that make floors slippery.
- Secure rugs so they don't slip.
- Wipe up spills promptly.
- Keep toys and other clutter off the floor.
- Check for other hazards on the floor, such as extension cords.

Lighting
- Illuminate corridors, stairwells, and closets, as well as rooms.
- Use night-lights or have flashlights available.
- Check for glare, which impairs good vision.

Stairs, bathrooms, kitchens, and furniture
- Install handrails on both sides of stairwells, if possible.
- Install grab bars and nonskid mats in the tub and shower.
- Organize cupboards and closets to minimize bending and reaching.
- Repair unsteady chairs and rickety tables.

FALLS CAN BE REDUCED!

Declining balance—like other age-related deterioration—can be addressed. Your doctor can help you pinpoint the source of the problem and suggest solutions. I hope you will ask for help if you're having any of these balance-related problems:

- If you have more than one fall per year that isn't related to a risky sport
- If fear of falling is curtailing your activities
- If you scored below "fair" on the balance test, or were concerned about the results of other tests in this chapter

Western scientists are beginning to appreciate what Eastern medical experts have known for centuries: that exercise can improve balance. One of my most exciting research findings was that women in our strength-training study improved an average 14 percent in balance scores. Meanwhile, the sedentary control group lost ground, with an 8 percent decline in balance during the year of the study.

I've been especially encouraged by the work of balance-training pioneers like Mary Tinetti, M.D., of Yale University, James Judge, M.D., of the University of Connecticut in Farmington; and John Campbell, M.D., of the University of Otago Medical School in New Zealand. They've shown that comprehensive interventions can make a dramatic difference.

For example, Mary Tinetti and her colleagues at Yale studied a group of 301 men and women, all age 70 or older, who had additional risk factors for falling. Half—the control group—received no special care. The rest were given intensive help to prevent falls. They learned exercises to improve their strength, balance, and coordination. Their medications were reviewed and adjusted if necessary. Investigators even visited their homes and suggested ways to eliminate hazards. At the end of the year, there had been 164 falls in the control group, but only 94 falls for those who'd been through the comprehensive program—a very significant reduction for a group at such high risk.

Other studies have obtained similar results. Even less ambitious interventions—just doing exercises, or simply correcting hazards in the home—make a significant difference. As we learn more, I expect to see new programs that are even more effective.

Balance is a fascinating subject that's finally getting the attention it deserves. We're learning that poor balance doesn't affect just the frail elderly; it's an issue for younger women too. We're all vulnerable to falls. But it's encouraging to learn how resilient our balance is—and that simple, enjoyable exercises make a real difference.

Smart Strategies
for Strong Bones

Calcium and Beyond

◆ ◆ ◆

G ood nutrition for bones involves a lot more than wearing a milk mustache or taking a calcium supplement. While calcium is essential, it's only part of the story. As you read this chapter, you'll learn about other nutrients that are also needed for optimal bone health. No matter what your food preferences—even if you're a vegan or lactose-intolerant—you can plan menus that support your bones. You'll gain other benefits too. It turns out that bone-friendly foods are also excellent for overall health.

THE CALCIUM CONNECTION

W e've known for more than two decades that there's a direct relationship between calcium consumption and bone strength. This shouldn't be surprising, because calcium is a significant part of our bone mass. It's especially important to get enough calcium when we're kids and young adults and still building bone. But we need it to help preserve our bone mass as we get older.

How much calcium do I need?

This sounds like a simple question. But it's been the subject of scientific debate for the past three decades. For years the National Academy of Sciences' Food and Nutrition Board had one set of guidelines for calcium—the famil-

ABOUT THE SCIENCE

Lessons from Podravia and Istra

Podravia and Istra are rural districts of the former Yugoslavia. In the late 1960s and early 1970s, a remarkably ambitious study of their populations yielded valuable information about calcium and bone.

The people of Podravia traditionally raise dairy cows, and their calcium intake is high. The people of Istra have the same genetic heritage, but that region grows more vegetables and grains, and calcium consumption typically is much lower. Velimir Matkovic, M.D., and colleagues from Medical School University of Zagreb in the former Yugoslavia wondered if these lifelong differences in eating habits would be reflected in their bones.

By checking diet histories from a sample of residents, the scientists learned that the average calcium intake of women in Podravia was 900 milligrams per day (mg/day); in Istra, the average was only 400 mg/day. Meanwhile, for six years, they tracked the hospital records of 159,446 people from Podravia and 174,250 from Istra, checking for fractures.

The result: Women in Istra, whose normal diet was low in calcium, experienced 225 hip fractures during the six-year period. But women from the dairy-producing district of Podravia had only 104 hip fractures. The results were published in the *American Journal of Clinical Nutrition* in 1979. Rereading this study today, when we know so much more about the importance of getting vitamin D and exercise along with calcium, I assume that women in both of these rural areas also benefited from a lifestyle that provided plenty of sun exposure and physical exertion.

iar RDAs (Recommended Dietary Allowances). But in 1994, a panel of experts from the National Institutes of Health (NIH) recommended higher levels of calcium consumption. In my first book, *Strong Women Stay Young*, I suggested that women follow the NIH guidelines. Those recommendations aimed at optimizing bone health, while the RDAs focused on the less ambitious goal of preventing deficiencies.

Meanwhile, thanks to continuing research, we were learning more about nutrition and health, including the relationship between calcium and bone. In 1997, the Food and Nutrition Board began to issue a new kind of recommendation called the Dietary Reference Intake (DRI). These are gradually replacing the RDAs, so you may see both terms for a while.

I agree with the new DRIs for calcium. They reflect the latest research; they're designed to optimize health. And they're practical. As you'll see from the menus at the end of this chapter, a woman who eats well can easily meet the DRI for calcium from her diet.

DIETARY REFERENCE INTAKE OF CALCIUM FOR WOMEN AND MEN	
AGE	CALCIUM DRI *(mg/day)*
Birth to 6 months	210
6 months to 1 year	270
1 to 3 years	500
4 to 8 years	800
9 to 18 years	1300
19 to 50 years	1000
51 to 70 years	1200
71 years and older	1200
Source: the National Academy of Sciences, 1997	

The best food sources of calcium

Dairy products top the list of calcium food sources. However, many nondairy foods contain significant amounts. Also, manufacturers now add calcium to processed foods like orange juice and breakfast cereal. Here's a quick overview of major food groups and their calcium content:

- **Dairy foods:** Most are high in calcium. If you wish to limit calories or fat, select low-fat or nonfat varieties.
- **Beans:** Soybeans and other beans are good sources of calcium. They're especially valuable for anyone who needs to limit calories or dairy foods.
- **Nuts:** Almonds and filberts are good calcium sources. However, they're high in fat and calories.
- **Vegetables:** Green leafy vegetables—including spinach, kale, broccoli, collards, and bok choy—are modest sources of calcium. They're also low in calories.
- **Fruit:** Certain fruits—especially oranges and raisins—provide modest amounts of calcium.
- **Meat, poultry, and fish:** Most contain little or no calcium, but there's an exception: fish consumed with the bones, such as canned salmon or sardines, is a very good source.
- **Grains:** Unless they're enriched, grains are not a particularly good source of calcium.

CALCIUM-RICH FOODS	SERVING SIZE	CALCIUM (in mg)
DAIRY PRODUCTS AND SOY MILK		
Milk (whole, low-fat, skim)	8 ounces	300
Protein-fortified milk	8 ounces	350
Yogurt (whole, low-fat, nonfat, flavored)	8 ounces	275–325
Protein-fortified yogurt	8 ounces	400–450

CALCIUM-RICH FOODS	SERVING SIZE	CALCIUM *(in mg)*
DAIRY PRODUCTS AND SOY MILK		
Hard cheeses high in calcium: cheddar, Swiss, Edam, Monterey Jack, provolone, Parmesan, Romano, part-skim mozzarella	1 ounce	200–300
Hard and soft cheeses with medium calcium levels: American, Gouda, Colby, whole-milk mozzarella, feta, fontina, blue cheese, Camembert	1 ounce	100–200
Soft cheeses lower in calcium: Brie, Neufchâtel, cream cheese (regular, low-fat)	1 ounce	20–50
Protein-fortified cream cheese	1 ounce	100
Cottage cheese (whole-milk, low-fat, nonfat)	½ cup	60–80
Ricotta (whole-milk, low-fat, nonfat)	½ cup	250–350
Ice cream and frozen yogurt (regular, low-fat, nonfat)	½ cup	70–120
Milk-based puddings and custards	½ cup	150
Soy milk (calcium-fortified)	8 ounces	200–300
Soy milk (not calcium-fortified)	8 ounces	10
SOY AND OTHER BEANS		
Soybeans: green boiled; edamame	½ cup	125
Soybeans: dry-roasted, soy nuts	½ cup	225
Tofu made with calcium sulfate	½ cup	250
Tofu made without calcium sulfate	½ cup	125
Tempeh	½ cup	77
Textured vegetable protein	½ cup	85
Miso paste	½ cup	91
Kidney beans, chickpeas, navy beans, pinto beans, green beans	½ cup	25–60

CALCIUM-RICH FOODS	SERVING SIZE	CALCIUM *(in mg)*
NUTS		
Almonds	1 ounce	75
Hazelnuts (filberts)	1 ounce	50
VEGETABLES		
Spinach, cooked	½ cup	125
Other leafy green vegetables (mustard greens, kale, bok choy, cabbage, sauerkraut), cooked	½ cup	50
Leafy green vegetables, raw	1 cup	50
Other vegetables (broccoli, green beans, squash), cooked	½ cup	30
Potatoes	1 medium	20
Rhubarb, cooked	½ cup	175
FRUITS		
Oranges, tangerines, grapefruit, mango, kiwi	1 medium	20–50
Orange juice (fresh–not calcium-fortified)	8 ounces	30
Prunes (dried)	10 dried	45
Raisins (regular or golden)	⅓ cup	25
FISH		
Fresh fish and seafood (bass, halibut, trout, clams, oysters, lobster)	3 ounces	40–70
Salmon (canned, with bones)	3 ounces	200
Sardines (canned, with bones)	2 sardines	100
Anchovy (canned, with bones)	3 ounces	125
CALCIUM-FORTIFIED FOODS (CHECK THE LABEL)		
Calcium-fortified orange juice	8 ounces	200–300
Calcium-fortified breakfast cereal and granola bars	1 cup	150–600
Calcium-fortified soy beverage	8 ounces	200–300

CALCIUM-RICH FOODS
OTHER FOODS
To learn the calcium content of foods that aren't listed, check the nutrition label if there is one. A standard source of nutrient data for professional nutritionists, which I used for the tables above, is *Bowes & Church's Food Values of Portions Commonly Used,* 17th edition, Jean A. T. Pennington, Ph.D., R.D. (Lippincott-Raven Publishers, 1998). This comprehensive reference book is available at most public libraries. Or search the online nutrition database of the United States Department of Agriculture (http://www.nal.usda.gov/fnic/cgi-bin/nut_search.pl).

What the labels mean

The nutrition labels on packaged foods use a special set of simplified standards—called the Daily Values (DVs)—based on the DRIs for middle-aged adults. Here are the Daily Values for the nutrients discussed in this chapter:

NUTRIENT	100% DV
Calcium	1000 milligrams
Vitamin D	400 international units
Vitamin K	80 micrograms
Vitamin C	60 milligrams
Potassium	3500 milligrams
Magnesium	400 milligrams

If the label on your calcium-fortified orange juice says that a serving has 30 percent of the DV of calcium, that's 30 percent of 1000 milligrams, or 300 milligrams of calcium.

How much calcium do I get from food?

Estimate your daily calcium consumption using the preceding table and the worksheet that follows. Don't be overly concerned about getting the num-

Do dairy foods and calcium actually cause osteoporosis?

This startling accusation—voiced by a few individuals and organizations—is based largely on studies of women in Africa and Asia. Despite their low consumption of milk and dairy products, these women are much less likely than their American counterparts to suffer from osteoporosis.

As you know from this book, experts agree that other factors are important for bone health too. African and Asian women may not have a high-calcium diet, but they beat the osteoporosis odds in other ways: Their diets include plenty of fruits and vegetables (plus soy in the case of Asians); they get much more exercise than most American women. They're also much less likely to drink or smoke. We'd all do well to follow their good example in those respects. But decades of research show that calcium and dairy foods really do help bone. And there's no credible evidence that they're harmful.

bers exactly right—a quick estimate is all you need. Your bones reflect your eating habits over months and years, not your consumption on a particular day.

- Think about everything you ate yesterday, or keep track today.
- Look at the table and count your servings of high-calcium foods (over 200 milligrams). Then count servings of foods that supply 100 to 199 milligrams, and servings of foods that provide less than 100 milligrams. Put the numbers in column B of the worksheet.
- Multiply by column A to fill in column C, and add it all up.

An even simpler approach is to visit the Web site of the Dairy Council of California (http://www.dairycouncilofca.org) and go to the section on families and kids, which has a quick interactive test.

FOODS	A APPROX. MG/SERVING	B # DAILY SERVINGS	A × B = C APPROX. TOTAL CALCIUM
Excellent calcium source (200 or more mg/serving)	300		
Good calcium source (100–199 mg/serving)	150		
Minor source (25–99 mg/serving)	50		
YOUR APPROXIMATE TOTAL DAILY CALCIUM INTAKE			
YOUR DRI (from table on page 101)			

Are you getting enough calcium? If so, congratulations! Nutrition surveys find that only about 10 percent of American women do. The average calcium intake is only 500 to 600 milligrams per day.

The calcium obstacles—and how to get around them

When I talk about nutrition and osteoporosis at lectures, women tell me, "I know I should get more calcium. But—" And then they describe an obstacle. It's almost always one of the three problems below. Fortunately, there are solutions.

"I don't like milk."

I always sympathize when a woman says this, because I feel the same way. Even though I rarely drink a glass of milk, I don't mind pouring it over breakfast cereal, or using it as a base for soups, shakes, or desserts. Milk is not the only dairy food that's loaded with calcium. Maybe you'd prefer yogurt or ice cream. You can grate hard cheese over pasta or use it instead of butter on bagels.

"I'm lactose-intolerant."

If you lack the enzyme needed to digest lactose (the sugar in milk), dairy foods may cause digestive problems. Sometimes the answer is as simple as cutting down the portion. Another approach is to add the enzyme (lactase) to food or to buy dairy products that already contain added lactase. Some lactose-intolerant women can tolerate cheese or yogurt made with live cultures (check the label).

"I don't eat animal products."

You can meet your calcium DRI from vegetable products if you select carefully. Choose plant-based foods that are high in calcium, such as tofu made with calcium sulfate (check the label).

Seven surprising (and simple) ways to boost your calcium intake

- Sweeten beverages, cereal, and home-baked breads and cakes with blackstrap molasses, which contains a whopping 172 milligrams of calcium per tablespoon. (Note: Regular molasses contains much less, but is still a fairly good source at 41 milligrams per tablespoon.)
- When you serve cottage cheese, stir in the whey—that watery liquid is rich in calcium. And while you're at it, consider a switch to ricotta, which has twice as much calcium per serving as cottage cheese.
- For snacks and casserole toppings, select high-calcium hard cheeses instead of softer or lower-calcium cheeses. For example, Swiss cheese has over 250 milligrams of calcium per ounce; mozzarella has only 150 to 200.
- Select protein-fortified dairy products. They're made with extra milk solids and contain significantly more calcium than nonfortified versions. For instance, ordinary cream cheese has 20 to 40 milligrams of calcium per serving. But a serving of protein-fortified nonfat cream cheese has 100 milligrams of calcium. Protein-fortified yogurt has 400 to 450 milligrams of calcium per serving, even more than the 275 to 325 milligrams of ordinary yogurt. Exact amounts vary considerably, so check labels.

- Look for calcium-fortified dairy products, which may contain significantly more calcium than nonfortified versions—up to 500 milligrams per cup.
- When you make soups and stews with meat or poultry, remove the bones *after* cooking instead of before. As these dishes simmer, some of the calcium leaches out of the bones, enriching the liquid. This effect is enhanced if the soup or stew includes acidic ingredients such as tomato, lemon, or vinegar. Similarly, if you're planning to grill, broil, or roast, select cuts of meat or poultry that include the bone. Marinate in wine, lemon juice, or vinegar, and include the leftover liquid—which is calcium-enriched—in the sauce or glaze.
- Buy tofu prepared with calcium sulfate. A ½ cup serving of tofu prepared with calcium sulfate has about 250 milligrams of calcium, twice as much as tofu prepared without calcium sulfate.

But is it bioavailable?

Calcium is so important to good health that you'd think the body would use every bit. But it doesn't. Most of us absorb only about a third of the calcium we consume. The rest is simply excreted. Certain foods, if eaten in excess, can adversely affect calcium absorption, or bioavailability. Here are some of the culprits—and how to avoid them. The key is moderation.

Fiber
Fiber keeps your digestive tract moving, which prevents constipation and wards off ailments like diverticulosis. But calcium bioavailability can suffer if you consume too much fiber. When food speeds through your intestines, there's not enough time to absorb all the calcium. Another issue: Fiber from the husks of grain contains phytic acid, which combines with calcium in the intestines and forms a compound that can't be absorbed.

These problems are unlikely to arise if you get your fiber from food. But unless your doctor has told you to *add* fiber to food (e.g., by sprinkling bran on cereal), it's best not to do so because it's easy to get too much that way.

Protein

Though adequate protein consumption is essential for strong bones, extremely high protein levels increase urinary excretion of calcium. While the American diet is rich in protein, it usually doesn't come close to this excess. But problems can develop when people follow unbalanced high-protein diets, or when they add protein supplements—such as powders and enriched drinks—to a diet that already has plenty of protein.

Caffeine

Caffeine is a diuretic. That means it increases the amount of urine you excrete—which also increases loss of calcium. Moderate amounts of caffeine don't have a significant effect. But keep your daily caffeine consumption under 400 milligrams—the equivalent of four cups of coffee. Other caffeine sources include tea, colas and certain other sodas, and some medications.

Sodium

Sodium in excess also increases urinary excretion of calcium. As the kidneys try to get rid of sodium, calcium is lost too. Many Americans consume too much sodium. The Food and Nutrition Board's Committee on Diet and Health recommends that adults consume no more than 2400 milligrams of sodium daily, but the average daily consumption in the United States is about 6000 milligrams per day. You can avoid the problem by using the saltshaker conservatively, and by limiting intake of highly processed foods and salty snacks.

Oxalates and oxalic acid

If you read about nutrition, perhaps you've seen warnings that oxalates and oxalic acid—compounds found in green leafy vegetables—unite with calcium during digestion and turn it into insoluble salts. You might wonder if it's wise to eat vegetables that contain oxalates. My answer is yes. While it's true that much of the calcium in leafy vegetables is unavailable because of oxalates, we still benefit from the remaining calcium and from many other nutrients in these vegetables.

Supplemental strategies

Nearly all experts agree that it's better to get nutrients from food than from pills. One very important reason is that we don't yet know all the beneficial

Can soda harm my bones?

You may have heard that the phosphorus in carbonated beverages interferes with calcium absorption. I'm not sure where this belief originated, but it's a myth.

Calcium metabolism can indeed suffer if you consume too much phosphorus. That's because both calcium and phosphorus require vitamin D for proper metabolism. An excess of phosphorus means that less vitamin D is available for processing calcium, so calcium absorption is reduced.

But soda is a negligible source of phosphorus in the typical American diet. Many sodas have no phosphorus at all—and even those that do contain phosphorus have modest amounts compared to other common foods.

For instance, there's no phosphorus at all in club soda or seltzer. Cola beverages have about 20 to 40 milligrams per 8-ounce serving, which is typical of sodas that contain phosphorus. To put that in perspective, consider that a glass of skim milk has over 200 milligrams of phosphorus, and half a cup of Kellogg's All-Bran has nearly 300. In other words, you'd have to drink more than two six-packs of Diet Coke to ingest as much phosphorus as you'd get from a modest serving of All-Bran and skim milk.

The *real* cause for concern about soda is that some people—especially children and teenagers—drink soda instead of milk, and as a result they don't consume enough calcium.

nutrients that foods contain. So women who rely on supplements may miss out. Also, it's much easier to overdo with supplements than with food. For instance, excess calcium can interfere with absorption of iron and zinc. You're not likely to consume enough calcium in your diet to cause a problem—but you might miscalculate with pills.

Yet another advantage of food is that calcium is more readily absorbed from dietary sources than from supplements. Typically, you get small amounts throughout the day—from breakfast cereal and milk, from a lunchtime yogurt shake, from a predinner cheese appetizer. Moreover, the calcium in food is dissolved and accompanied by natural sugars, which aid absorption. A friend told me an amusing story:

> *I talked to my doctor about osteoporosis at my last checkup. She questioned me about my diet, and told me I should be getting more calcium. I'd been reading about supplements and knew bioavailability was an issue. So I asked if there was a brand of calcium supplements available in liquid form with natural sugars. She said, "Yes. It's called milk."*

Because of all these advantages, I urge you to make a strong effort to increase your consumption of calcium-rich foods. This chapter offers many ideas. But if it just isn't possible for you to meet the calcium DRI by diet alone, the next best approach is to take a supplement.

Here's my strategy for getting the most out of supplements:

Step 1: Calculate how much extra calcium you need.
Use the worksheet or Web address I gave you earlier (see pages 106–7) to figure out how much calcium you get, and calculate your deficit. That's how much extra you need. Check the supplement label to find out how much elemental calcium (i.e., pure calcium) it provides. Most pills contain 200 to 500 milligrams of elemental calcium. There's no need to go above your DRI. Indeed, you might have digestive problems if you do.

Step 2: Decide what kind of supplement to take.
The two most widely used supplements are:

- **Calcium carbonate:** This is the most common kind of calcium supplement. It's available in many forms, including capsules, chewable tablets, and caramel chews, as well as in antacids like Tums. Most calcium carbonate supplements supply around 200 to 500 milligrams of elemental calcium per pill. Calcium carbonate requires acid to dissolve and be absorbed efficiently. Some women—especially older women—do not produce much stomach acid between

What about other kinds of calcium supplements?

If you browse the shelves of a drugstore or a health food store, you'll find a bewildering array of options. Here are a few suggestions:

- Avoid supplements made from calcium phosphate. If you're like most women, you get plenty of phosphorus from your diet—and an excess can interfere with calcium metabolism.
- Skip calcium gluconate and calcium lactate supplements. They contain much less calcium per tablet than conventional supplements, so they're usually less convenient and more costly than calcium carbonate or calcium citrate.
- Be cautious about calcium supplements made from oyster shells or bonemeal. Though the situation has improved, in the past some of these "natural" supplements also contained toxic contaminants, such as lead.
- Don't pay extra for "chelated" calcium supplements. There's no good scientific evidence that they're more absorbable or otherwise superior.

meals. So it's important to take the supplement at mealtime, when your stomach secretes extra acid.

- **Calcium citrate:** New evidence suggests that calcium citrate may be more readily absorbed than calcium carbonate. And there's a convenience advantage: Since calcium citrate contains acid, it doesn't require stomach acid for absorption. So you can take it at any time of day, whether or not you've just eaten. However, this type of supplement is usually more expensive than calcium carbonate. Also, since each pill contains just 200 or 300 milligrams of elemental calcium, you may need to take more pills.

The bottom line: Either kind of supplement is fine—what's best is whatever your body tolerates best. Select a brand that also contains 400 IU of vitamin D, unless you're getting vitamin D from other sources such as a multivitamin supplement. Vitamin D will help you absorb the calcium.

Step 3: Figure out how to get the most out of your supplements.

Some people experience mild indigestion from calcium supplements, including bloating, constipation, or loose bowels. Here are a few suggestions for avoiding problems—and getting the most from a calcium supplement:

- Since the body can't readily absorb large doses of calcium (over 500 milligrams) at once, spread your calcium consumption—both food and supplements—over the day. For example, if most of your daily calcium intake comes from two supplements plus breakfast cereal with milk, take one supplement in the afternoon and the other in the evening.
- If you take just one tablet per day, take it in the evening—after dinner (if it's calcium carbonate) or before bedtime (if it's calcium citrate). Your digestive system moves more slowly at night, which will allow the calcium and vitamin D extra time to be absorbed.
- If you experience indigestion, try taking the supplement at another time. Or divide the tablet and take half at a different time. Or switch to the other type of supplement—go to carbonate if you are using citrate, and vice versa.
- If you buy a brand that hasn't met USP (United States Pharmacopoeia) standards, give it the vinegar test to make sure it dissolves properly: Place one tablet in a cup filled with vinegar, and stir every five minutes. If the tablet doesn't disintegrate in thirty minutes, it probably won't disintegrate in your stomach either, so switch to another supplement. Discard the vinegar after the test.

VITAL VITAMIN D

Many women don't realize that vitamin D is just as important as calcium for strong bones—if not *more* important. Without this essential vitamin, our bodies can't use calcium properly. Vitamin D not only

New ways to get extra calcium

I don't enjoy milk as a beverage—but I love orange juice. So I was delighted when calcium-enriched orange juice appeared in my local supermarket. I prefer drinking juice to taking a pill: I know the calcium is already dissolved and is accompanied by sugars from the juice, which help with calcium absorption. Also, I get other important nutrients—vitamin C and potassium—simultaneously. Manufacturers now add calcium to other foods, such as breakfast cereal, granola bars, and soy beverages. And they've devised other ingenious ways to help us get the calcium we need: chewy candies that taste like caramels, chewing gum, and a powder that can be added to water or juice to create a sparkling beverage. Undoubtedly there will be more options in the future.

A few important cautions about calcium-enriched foods:

• Check the label to make sure you're getting the amount of calcium and vitamin D you need.
• Remember that these are medications. Keep them away from children, who may be tempted by what look like tasty treats.
• Don't get all your calcium from orange juice and candy. Foods that are high in calcium also contain other important nutrients, such as protein. This is particularly important for children, who need to establish healthy eating habits, and for the elderly, who may not get sufficient protein.

helps with calcium absorption, it also aids in the biochemical process by which calcium turns into bone. In fact, when you read the fine print in scientific studies of fractures and calcium supplements, the only research showing reductions in fractures are studies where calcium was combined with vitamin D!

We get vitamin D from two sources: diet (including supplements) and sun exposure. The typical American lifestyle provides enough vitamin

D for young women. But after age 50, our bodies have greater difficulty absorbing this essential vitamin from food and producing it from sun exposure. So even if our habits remain the same, deficiencies may become a problem.

ABOUT THE SCIENCE

Vitamin D reduces fractures

In the late 1980s and early 1990s, research on calcium supplements came up with disappointing results: taking supplements didn't reduce fractures. At the same time, scientists were learning more about the importance of vitamin D for bone. My colleague Bess Dawson-Hughes, M.D., and associates at Tufts wondered if adding vitamin D to calcium supplements would make a difference.

For three years the team tracked the bone health of 389 men and women age 65 and up. About half of the volunteers were given a daily supplement containing 500 milligrams of calcium and 700 IU of vitamin D; the rest received a placebo. During the three years, men and women in the two groups were about equally likely to fall. Thirteen percent of those who weren't taking the supplement suffered a fracture. But among those who received vitamin D, only 6 percent broke a bone. This benefit is comparable to the effects of hormone replacement therapy and other medications used to treat osteoporosis.

Another study, by Murray Tilyard, M.D., at the University of Otago in New Zealand, tracked 622 postmenopausal women with at least one vertebral fracture. Half received vitamin D supplements without added calcium; the others were given calcium only. During three years of follow-up, there were twenty-four additional fractures in the calcium group, but only eleven fractures in the group that took vitamin D—an impressive 60 percent reduction!

Vitamin D and food

The DRIs for vitamin D increase as we get older. Most women get 100 to 200 IU per day in their diet. That's enough for young women (who also get vitamin D from sun exposure)—but it's well under the higher DRI for those over 50.

VITAMIN D REQUIREMENTS FOR WOMEN AND MEN	
AGE	DRI *In international units and micrograms (mcg) equivalent 40 IU = 1 mcg*
Birth to age 50	200 IU or 5 mcg
51 to 70	400 IU or 10 mcg
71 and older	600 IU or 15 mcg
Source: the National Academy of Sciences, 1997	

The problem is that few foods naturally contain significant amounts of vitamin D. The best sources are cold saltwater fish and other seafood, like salmon, halibut, herring, tuna, Atlantic mackerel, oysters, and shrimp. The liver and oil from these fish are extremely high in vitamin D. Some mushrooms are also good sources, including shiitakes and morels.

Because this vitamin is so important, a committee of the American Medical Association recommended in 1957 that milk be fortified with 400 IU of vitamin D per quart. This requirement has been mandated by the federal government ever since. Vitamin D is also added to some fortified cereals and to many calcium supplements.

Vitamin D and the sun

Our other source of vitamin D is the sun. Special cells in our skin produce vitamin D when they're activated by ultraviolet light. A young woman who spends part of her day outdoors in the summer can get all the vitamin D she needs from the sun. But this is much more difficult for older women. If a 65-year-old woman and her 35-year old daughter take a ten-minute walk on a sunny day, the mother's skin will manufacture only a third of the amount of vitamin D that her daughter's does. To make matters worse, the angle of the sun's rays changes in the winter, and in many parts of the country even a sunny day doesn't provide the necessary stimulation for our skin cells. If you live in an area that's far enough north for snow, you probably don't get enough vitamin D during the winter. That's not a serious problem for healthy young women, whose bodies can store vitamin D through the winter. Even so, several studies have shown that bone density drops slowly through the winter, reaching a low point in late spring. The loss can amount to 3 or 4 percent.

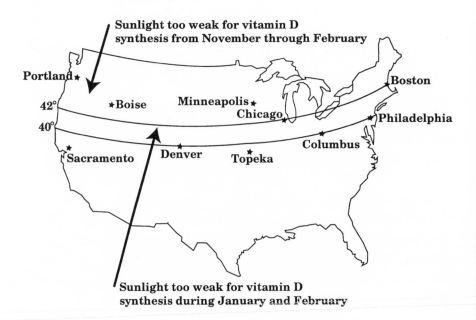

How to be sure you get enough

Unless you eat a lot of fish, or regularly consume vitamin D–fortified foods, chances are that you get less than the DRI from your diet. If you're 50 or younger and spend time outdoors, sun exposure can compensate. But if you're older, you may need more.

Here are my recommendations:

If you're 50 or younger and don't have osteopenia or osteoporosis:

If your diet is healthy and you spend time outdoors, you probably get enough vitamin D, so you don't need to take a supplement. However, if you're taking a calcium supplement, I suggest you select one that has added vitamin D to help absorption.

A guide to safe sun exposure

Sun exposure helps our bodies produce vitamin D—but excess sun also can cause dry skin, wrinkles, age spots, and skin cancer. When you wear sunscreen, you block the beneficial rays as well as the harmful ones. Fortunately, it's possible to avoid the dangers without giving up the benefits. Here's how:

- Always protect the delicate skin on your face by wearing sunscreen with an SPF of at least 15.
- Expose your arms and legs to the sun for ten to fifteen minutes per day, preferably in the middle of the day when the sun is high in the sky.
- After fifteen minutes, put on sunscreen to protect all exposed skin if you plan to stay out in the sun for any greater length of time.

*If you're between 51 and 70 and don't have
osteopenia or osteoporosis:*
Get daily sun exposure during the summer. In the fall, winter, and spring,
take a vitamin D supplement.

*If you're older than 70, or if you have
osteopenia or osteoporosis:*
Take a vitamin D supplement year round.

THE NEWEST BONE NUTRIENTS

Calcium and vitamin D are the most important nutrients for bone—and the ones we know the most about. However, we're beginning to learn that other vitamins and minerals play a much more significant role than previously realized.

Magnesium

Magnesium is one of the minerals that make up bone—and it's also important for many chemical reactions in the body, including conduction of nerve impulses to the heart and other parts of the body.

Research indicates that people whose diets are rich in magnesium have denser bones. However, evidence of magnesium bone benefits isn't nearly as strong for supplements. A few studies in older women suggested that supplements might help, but these investigations had methodological flaws so the results are not conclusive. I look forward to further research that finally provides clear answers.

Some calcium supplements contain magnesium as well as vitamin D. Though there's no harm in adding magnesium, I don't think we have sufficient data to know that it's helpful. Instead, I urge you to think of magnesium as yet another important benefit of a diet that includes plenty of fruits and vegetables and whole grains. Most women don't get quite as much magnesium as they should. The DRI for magnesium is 320 milligrams per day for women, but the average actual intake is only around 250 to 300 per day. Though this is a small deficit, it might contribute to osteoporosis.

You can easily increase your consumption of magnesium, because it's contained in so many healthy foods. Among the best sources are potatoes, seeds, nuts, legumes, and whole grains (most of the magnesium is in the husk and germ). Magnesium is also found in chlorophyll, so any dark green vegetable—romaine lettuce, spinach, kale—contains a good supply. The darker the color, the better. Other good sources are bananas, oranges, and tomatoes.

Potassium

Potassium is the latest nutrient with research-proven benefits for bone. Katherine Tucker's nutritional research on Framingham Heart study participants found that women whose diet is high in potassium have denser bones in their spine and hip; one other study has documented the same effect. The likely reason: Potassium contributes to the proper acid balance in the blood, so the body doesn't need to draw calcium from the skeleton for this purpose. Potassium serves us in other ways: it's needed for proper fluid balance in our bodies, for conduction of nerve impulses, and for muscle contractions.

There's no DRI for potassium, but the Daily Value (DV)—what's used for food labels—is 3500 milligrams. In Dr. Tucker's study, a woman's diet was considered high in potassium if she consumed 3500 to 6000 milligrams per day. That's not difficult to do if you eat plenty of fruits—especially oranges and bananas—and vegetables. Dairy products contain moderate amounts of potassium. So far there's no research supporting the use of potassium supplements for bone.

Vitamin K

Vitamin K is required for blood clotting and also contributes to production of collagen, a component of cartilage, connective tissue, and bone. Women typically consume about 70 micrograms daily of vitamin K, about what's currently recommended. However, I suspect the new DRIs will be slightly higher. New research suggests that middle-aged and older women who consume at least 110 micrograms of vitamin K per day have 30 percent fewer hip fractures than those who merely get the average amount. The reason isn't yet clear. We know that vitamin K contributes to production of osteocalcin, a protein critical for bone formation. But the bone benefits that apparently come from vitamin K might be at least partly caused by other nutrients present in foods that are high in this vitamin.

If you eat plenty of fruits and vegetables, it's easy to boost your vitamin K intake to 110 micrograms—just one portion of broccoli, cauliflower, brussels sprouts, spinach, or collard greens contains more than that amount. Other good sources include soy products, strawberries, some vegetable oils (soybean, canola, and olive), and liver. Since this is a fat-soluble vitamin, it's helpful to consume vitamin K–rich foods with a little fat or oil.

I don't recommend taking vitamin K supplements. Food is a better source because of all its additional nutrients.

Vitamin C

Vitamin C is an antioxidant. That means it combats the process of oxidation, which is a major factor in the aging of our bodies. This important vitamin keeps our skin, eyes, and gums healthy; it helps ward off infection. And vitamin C also appears to play an important role in collagen production—the first step in bone formation.

Most women get around 70 milligrams per day, slightly above the current recommendation of 60 milligrams per day. However, there's evidence that women whose diet contains more vitamin C have better bones. The best sources are citrus fruits. But other fruits (especially bananas, cantaloupe, and strawberries) and some vegetables (including peppers, broccoli, asparagus, cauliflower, tomatoes, and potatoes) also contain significant amounts. With all those luscious options, it's easy to get plenty of vitamin C from food.

Other nutrients

I frequently see calcium supplements that add not only vitamin D but also a whole chemistry set of trace elements like silicon, manganese, copper, zinc, and boron. While all are important for bone development and for general health, there's absolutely no evidence that supplementation with these nutrients will provide any benefit for the bones of a healthy woman. I urge you to approach vitamin and mineral supplements with caution until safety and efficacy have been proven in careful scientific research. Food is still our best source of nutrients—we're learning more about its riches every day.

SOY STRATEGIES

Some of the most exciting nutritional research on bone involves soy. Soybeans are a staple in Asian countries. But until recently, soy products were consumed mainly by vegetarians in the United States. The rest of us didn't know what we were missing! Soybeans are a great source of protein, but unlike animal products, they're free of cholesterol and relatively low in fat. Once you get acquainted with them, they're delicious.

We're beginning to appreciate another characteristic of soy: it's rich in daidzein and genistein, two major types of isoflavone, which is a form of phytoestrogen. In other words, soy contains compounds that act like weak estrogens in the body. Animal research has already shown that a diet high in soy can improve bone—at least in rodents. One reason could be that osteoblasts (the cells that build bone) have receptors for genistein and other isoflavones. Also, isoflavones may inhibit bone breakdown. Soy products contain other nutrients, such as vitamin K, which may contribute as well.

In Chapter 9, on medication, I'll discuss a synthetic isoflavone called ipriflavone that has been widely tested in humans. But so far there's been only one well-designed scientific report on the effects of soy-based nutritional supplements on people. A 1998 University of Illinois study followed 66 postmenopausal women for six months to see if soy protein that contained various amounts of isoflavone would improve their bone density. A third of the women received a high dose of isoflavone, a third received a medium dose, and a control group was given a placebo. Results were promising, though not dramatic. The control group had a .5 percent decline in bone density, as is normal in untreated postmenopausal women. Those who took the medium dose of isoflavone had no gain or loss of bone. The women who consumed the high dose showed no improvement in bone density at the hip, but bone density in the spine increased by an average 2.25 percent.

Since soy has many health-promoting qualities, I encourage you to add it to your diet. But until there's more data to confirm that soy supplements are safe and effective, I don't recommend them.

Putting soy on your menu

Are you convinced that soy is good for you—but uncertain what to buy or how to prepare it? Below is a quick guide. Supermarkets carry an increasing variety of soy products. They're also found at health food stores and at groceries that sell Asian food. Note: Some soy products—but not all—are excellent calcium sources, so read the labels carefully. For more information about soy products—and lots of recipes—visit the Web site of the Indiana Soybean Board: http://www.soyfoods.com.

- **Soy milk** is the liquid from soybeans. It's often sold with added flavor and sweeteners. If you don't drink regular milk, substitute plain soy milk that's fortified with calcium.
- **Tofu** is the soy equivalent of firm cottage cheese. Indeed, it has a bland dairylike taste, something like a soft, very mild cheese. Because tofu has so little flavor of its own, it's very versatile. Try substituting small cubes of tofu for all or half of the meat or poultry in your favorite stir-fry, casserole, or salad.
- **Tempeh** is a fermented form of soybean. It's firmer than tofu, with a delicious nutty flavor. You can buy tempeh in flat blocks, ready to grill or to dice and stir-fry.
- **Soy nuts** are roasted soybeans. They can be eaten as snacks or added to salads.
- **Textured vegetable protein** (TVP) is soy protein. It's sold plain in dry form; you can add it to casseroles as you would add cooked hamburger crumbles. TVP is usually the main ingredient in frozen vegetarian burgers and many vegetarian convenience foods, such as vegetarian sausage or chili mixes.
- **Edamame** are soybeans steamed or boiled in the pod, a favorite of mine. They make a sweet and delicious addition to salad, or can be eaten like nuts as an appetizer. At my local supermarket, which carries a good selection of Japanese foods, they're sold in bags in the frozen vegetable section. I steam them for a few minutes, let them cool, then strip the pod off and eat them up!

FIVE WAYS TO FEED YOUR BONES

I know that some women have trouble consuming enough calcium and other bone-boosting nutrients. But with a little planning, it's really not that difficult. Here are five simple daily menus that are designed to show how easy it is for women with a variety of food preferences and nutritional concerns to eat well. Each menu provides at least 1200 milligrams of calcium, plus ample amounts of fruits, vegetables, whole grains, and soy—which means you're getting all the nutrients you need for strong bones. Some of the menus are lower in calories, some higher. Use them as a starting point for devising meals that match your own food preferences and caloric needs.

"I enjoy milk and have no dietary restrictions."

If you like milk, you can easily meet your calcium DRI with a well-balanced diet that includes two or three glasses of milk.

Meal	Menu	Calcium (mg)	Calories
Breakfast	¾ cup whole-grain fortified cereal	250	110
	1 cup milk (1% fat)	300	102
	½ cup raspberries	13	30
	1 slice cinnamon-raisin toast	12	86
	1 Tbs jam	4	48
Lunch	1 cup minestrone soup	60	107
	Grilled chicken sandwich		
	1 whole-wheat roll	30	75
	3 oz grilled chicken	13	148
	lettuce, tomato (2 slices)	10	11
	2 tsp mayonnaise	0	66
	1 cup chocolate milk (1% fat)	287	158
	1 medium banana	7	105

Continued

MEAL	MENU (mg)	CALCIUM	CALORIES
Dinner	6 oz trout, grilled	146	256
	1 medium baked potato	20	220
	1 Tbs sour cream	14	26
	Salad		
	½ cup romaine	10	4
	½ cup spinach	28	6
	½ medium tomato	3	13
	½ cup cucumber	7	7
	1 oz cheddar cheese	204	114
	¼ cup tofu, crumbled	129	91
	1 Tbs creamy Italian dressing	0	55
Snack	½ cup ice cream	72	143

Totals

Calcium: 1619 mg

Calories: 1981

Fruit and vegetable servings: 6

Soy servings: 1

"I'm watching my weight."

Some dairy foods are high in fat—but not all. If you're watching your weight, be sure to select nonfat or low-fat versions of milk, yogurt, and other dairy foods. Dark green leafy vegetables boost calcium without weighing down the calorie count.

Meal	Menu	Calcium (mg)	Calories
Breakfast	Egg white omelet		
	½ cup egg whites	8	74
	1 oz low-fat cheddar cheese	118	49
	½ cup chopped broccoli	21	12
	1 tsp safflower oil	0	41
	1 slice whole-wheat bread	20	69
	1 cup skim milk	302	86
Lunch	Salad		
	½ cup romaine	10	4
	½ cup spinach	28	6
	½ cup peppers	5	14
	½ medium carrot	10	15
	½ cup chickpeas	38	143
	½ apple	5	40
	2 Tbs low-fat dressing	0	70
	2 oz oat-bran pita bread	100	130
Dinner	Turkey and vegetable pasta		
	1 cup pasta	10	197
	2 oz diced turkey	11	90
	½ cup low-fat ricotta cheese	337	171
	½ cup spinach	122	21
	½ medium tomato	3	13
	1 shiitake mushroom	1	10
	½ Tbs grated Parmesan cheese	34	12
Snack	½ cup vanilla pudding with low-fat soy milk	150	153

Totals

Calcium: 1333 mg   Fruit and vegetable servings: 5

Calories: 1420   Soy servings: 1

"I don't like milk!"

Lots of women don't like to drink milk. But they're happy to tuck other enjoyable dairy foods into their meals throughout the day.

MEAL	MENU	CALCIUM (mg)	CALORIES
Breakfast	Waffle stack		
	2 multigrain waffles	40	181
	½ cup yogurt	200	70
	½ cup blueberries	4	40
	1 Tbs maple syrup	13	52
	1 cup fresh-squeezed orange juice	27	112
Lunch	Turkey-tofu sandwich		
	1 oz turkey breast	5	25
	¼ cup sliced tofu	129	91
	lettuce, tomato (2 slices)	10	11
	2 slices whole-wheat bread	40	138
	2 kosher dill pickle spears	36	8
	1 Tbs mayonnaise	0	100
	1 orange	52	60
Dinner	Chef's salad		
	1 cup Bibb lettuce	20	8
	1 cup spinach	56	12
	½ cucumber	7	7
	½ carrot	10	15
	½ tomato	3	13
	1 oz Monterey Jack cheese	212	106
	2 oz baked ham	5	83
	1 Tbs dressing	0	55

Continued

Meal	Menu	Calcium (mg)	Calories
	1 cup clam chowder	40	200
	1 medium piece corn bread	161	176
	1 tsp butter	1	36
Snack	Banana-pineapple smoothie		
	½ cup yogurt	200	70
	½ banana	4	52
	½ cup pineapple juice	21	70

Totals

Calcium: 1296 mg

Calories: 1791

Fruit and vegetable servings: 9

Soy servings: 1

Ten ways to sneak high-calcium dairy foods into your diet if you don't like milk

- For breakfast, melt hard cheese onto toast or bagel. Or use protein-enriched nonfat cream cheese.
- Use yogurt in salad dressings.
- Top vegetables with grated cheese instead of butter.
- Include sliced cheese on sandwiches.
- Add cheese to pasta, salads, soups, and casseroles.
- Serve ice cream, frozen yogurt, or milk-based pudding for desserts.
- Make shakes and smoothies for snacks.
- Add milk powder to soups and casseroles.
- Serve pasta dishes like ricotta ravioli, lasagna with cheese layers, and macaroni and cheese.
- Drink coffee or espresso with steamed milk.

"I'm lactose intolerant—dairy foods don't agree with me."

No doubt about it, lactose intolerance adds to the challenge of getting all the calcium you need. But if you select carefully—and take advantage of high-calcium vegetables and fish—you can do it.

Meal	Menu	Calcium (mg)	Calories
Breakfast	½ medium grapefruit	15	39
	1 cup cooked oatmeal	19	145
	⅓ cup raisins	25	150
	1 cup soy milk	300	110
Lunch	Bean and chicken burritto		
	½ cup black beans	23	113
	2 oz chicken	9	99
	½ cup brown rice	10	109
	2 Tbs tomato salsa	10	10
	1 medium tortilla	44	56
	Fruit salad		
	¼ cup cantaloupe	5	14
	¼ cup honeydew	3	15
	¼ cup strawberries	11	5
	1 oz walnuts	16	172
	½ cup oats and honey granola	61	219
Dinner	6 oz salmon (canned with bones)	424	240
	½ cup butternut squash	42	41
	½ cup brussels sprouts	28	30
	½ cup spinach pasta	42	182
	½ cup green beans	29	22
Snack	1 orange	52	60
	½ cup custard made with soy milk	150	140

Continued

Totals
Calcium: 1318 mg
Calories: 1971
Fruit and vegetable servings: 7
Soy servings: 2

"I'm a vegan."

Vegans consume no animal products at all, which rules out dairy foods. But it's still possible to get enough calcium in your diet. Some suggestions:

- Eat dark green leafy vegetables every day.
- Add tofu to casseroles, lasagnas, salads, and so on.
- Select calcium-fortified soy drinks, orange juice, and cereals.

Meal	Menu	Calcium (mg)	Calories
Breakfast	3½ inch sesame seed bagel	53	195
	1 Tbs peanut butter	6	95
	1 cup freshly squeezed grapefruit juice	22	96
Lunch	Hummus sandwich		
	½ cup hummus	61	210
	2 slices whole-wheat bread	40	138
	½ cup sprouts	5	5
	1 medium apple	10	81
	1 oz sunflower seeds, dried	34	160
	1 cup vanilla soy milk	300	110
Dinner	Vegetable-rice stir-fry		
	1 cup long-grain brown rice, enriched	20	216
	½ cup broccoli	21	12
	½ cup bok choy	11	13
	½ cup kale	47	21

Continued

Meal	Menu	Calcium (mg)	Calories
	½ cup tofu	258	182
	1 oz almonds	80	166
	⅓ cup golden raisins	26	151
	1 Tbs tamari soy sauce	4	12
	2 tsp olive oil	0	83
Snack	¼ cup edamame	65	63
	½ mango	10	67
	1 cup chocolate soy milk	300	110

Totals

Calcium: 1374 mg

Calories: 2187

Fruit and vegetable servings: 8

Soy servings: 3

A healthy diet—one that contains sufficient calcium and vitamin D as well as plenty of fruits and vegetables—can reduce your risk of bone fractures by an impressive 30 to 40 percent. What's more, such a diet also decreases your risk for heart disease, diabetes, and other chronic ailments. Of course, it's best to start eating well early in life. But even if it's too late for that, you can make meaningful improvements if you begin now. Good nutrition doesn't require elaborate cooking. With a little savvy planning, you can boost the nutritional power of your diet without spending a lot of extra time. And it will taste terrific too!

Nutrition information resources

Organization

American Dietetic Association (ADA)

216 West Jackson Boulevard; Chicago, IL 60606-6995; 800/366-1655
http://www.eatright.org

Newsletter and books

Tufts University Health & Nutrition Newsletter
PO Box 420235; Palm Coast, FL 32142-0235; 800/274-7581
http://www.healthletter.tufts.edu

The Wellness Encyclopedia of Food and Nutrition, by Sheldon Margen,
M.D., and the editors of the University of California at Berkeley
Wellness Letter (Rebus, 1992)

Nancy Clark's Sport Nutrition Guidebook, by Nancy Clark, M.S., R.D.
(Human Kinetics, 1996)

Jane Brody's Good Food Book, by Jane Brody (Bantam, 1987)

Online resources

Tufts University Nutrition Navigator (http://navigator.tufts.edu) has
links to hundreds of nutrition and health resources.

USDA Nutrient Database (http://www.nal.usda.gov/fnic/) has
detailed nutritional information about foods.

Cyberdiet (http://www.cyberdiet.com) offers nutrition information,
recipes, assessment tools, and a variety of support groups.

CHAPTER 8

Bone-Boosting
Workouts

◆ ◆ ◆

Our bones are slowly shaped by the forces they withstand. The more active we are, the stronger our bones will be. These changes don't happen quickly—they're not the result of a single walk or a tennis match. But if we walk daily, or if we play tennis regularly, the pounding of our feet against the pavement or our racket arm against the ball will stimulate our bones. Women who exercise throughout their lives have stronger bones than their sedentary counterparts. But it's never too late to start!

This chapter presents a comprehensive exercise program, based on the latest scientific information, designed specifically to defend against osteoporosis and falls. The program was developed with the assistance of my colleague Jennifer Layne, M.S., C.S.C.S.—an extraordinarily knowledgeable and talented trainer who has extensive experience working with men and women affected by osteoporosis. You'll see her special notes after each exercise—please consider her your personal trainer.

The *Strong Women, Strong Bones* exercise program requires as little as half an hour per day. This tiny investment of time produces truly remarkable effects. You'll strengthen your bones and muscles. Your balance will improve, adding to your protection from fractures. And that's not all. The beauty of physical activity is that it has numerous beneficial side effects! People who get regular exercise reduce their risk for many chronic diseases associated with aging. There are much more immediate benefits too. As you become fitter, your cardiovascular system will be healthier, so you'll have more energy. Your body will be leaner, so you'll find weight control easier—muscle burns more calories than fat. Many women find that exercise improves their mood and self-esteem as well. These effects are evident very quickly, before your bones have time to change. So you'll feel healthier and happier right from the start.

ELEMENTS OF THE *STRONG WOMEN, STRONG BONES* EXERCISE PROGRAM

The best program for osteoporosis is one that combines five different types of exercise. Weight-bearing aerobic exercise, high-impact activities, and strength training help build bone. Just as important are exercises that address balance and flexibility. The *Strong Women, Strong Bones* program includes all of these elements.

Weight-bearing aerobic activity

Weight-bearing activities create impact on bone each time your feet hit the ground. The bones of your hip and spine benefit particularly from these exercises.

The *Strong Women, Strong Bones* exercise program encourages you to gradually increase the intensity as well as the duration of weight-bearing aerobic exercise. When you're standing or strolling, the impact on your bones is about equal to your body weight. But if you walk briskly or jog, the forces acting on your skeleton increase to double or triple your body weight. And there's a bonus: extra aerobic effort will improve your cardiovascular fitness.

High-impact exercises

Women who walk regularly have stronger bones than sedentary women. But the gentle stimulation of walking takes decades to produce effects. Researchers have found that high-impact activities—such as tennis, volleyball, basketball, jumping rope, and vertical jumping—can improve bone much more quickly. During these exercises, your bones are subjected to forces that are three to six times greater than your body weight. Of course, the downside of these forces is that they can be hard on your joints. High-impact activities aren't safe for everyone. I'll give you the necessary cautions and explain how to get the benefits without the problems.

Strength training

My research, published in the *Journal of the American Medical Association* in 1994, showed that strength training just twice a week dramatically cuts the risk of fractures for postmenopausal women. After a year, participants gained bone in their hip and spine; they became stronger and their balance improved.

Numerous other studies have confirmed the finding that strength training builds bone. How does it work? Muscles are attached to bones by tendons. As the muscles contract, they tug against the bones. This stimulates the bones to grow. The stronger the muscles, the more powerful the stimulation they provide. By building stronger muscles, strength training helps your bones even between workouts.

The strength-training exercises in this book promote general health and fitness, but they were selected with osteoporosis in mind. Several moves target muscles in the hip, spine and arms—areas particularly vulnerable to fractures. Other exercises were chosen for their balance benefits.

Balance training

Balance training doesn't increase bone density. However, it protects whatever bone we have by preventing falls. If you're under age 50, you probably have good balance. Still, these exercises are beneficial. First, they're a fun way to cool down after a workout. I enjoy doing balance exercises with my kids, because they love them too. Also, I strongly believe that if we work our balance systems when we're younger, we can avoid (or at least minimize) the usual deterioration in balance as we get older.

Stretching

Stretching is an important component of any well-rounded exercise program. If you have strong, flexible joints, all physical activities will be easier and more enjoyable—and you're less likely to suffer injuries. If you're concerned about osteoporosis, an added benefit is that stretching improves overall flexibility. That's helpful for preventing falls.

A twelve-week progressive program

If you're physically active now, you may already be doing some of the exercises I suggest. That's great! You'll learn how to build upon this excellent foundation. If you're sedentary, this program will gently ease you into a more active lifestyle. During the first few weeks, your workouts will take less than half an hour. As your fitness improves, you'll add exercises. At the end of twelve weeks, you'll be exercising for as little as forty minutes per day and getting the full bone benefits of this program.

You'll start with just three fifteen-minute sessions of weight-bearing aerobic activity plus four strengthening exercises done three times a week. Each workout will include a few balance exercises and stretches to cool down. If you're premenopausal and healthy, you'll also do vertical jumps—a two-minute exercise with significant benefits for bone. Depending on your preferred schedule for this initial period, your entire workout will take twenty to forty minutes and will be done three to six times per week.

By the end of twelve weeks, you'll be doing thirty minutes of weight-bearing aerobic exercise and a total of ten strengthening exercises. Each workout will include balancing exercises and stretches, and possibly vertical jumping as well. You can complete these exercises in six forty-minute workouts per week or, if you prefer, you can schedule three longer workouts.

BEFORE YOU BEGIN

Many women skip medical checkups. They're busy; they're feeling fine and don't see the need; they worry about the expense or fear bad news. But routine physical examinations are an essential part of staying healthy—they can uncover serious medical problems long before symptoms appear, when treatment is most effective. If you haven't had a checkup for a year or more, please make an appointment. This is especially important if you're at risk for osteoporosis.

The exercise programs in this book are safe for nearly everyone. However, some women—including those with a history of fractures—need to talk to a doctor before increasing their physical activity. Take the PAR-Q (Physical Activity Readiness Questionnaire) to see if this caution applies to

Physical Activity Readiness
Questionnare—PAR-Q
(revised 1994)

PAR-Q & YOU
(A Questionnaire for People Aged 15 to 69)

Regular physical activity is fun and healthy, and increasingly more people are starting to become more active every day. Being more active is very safe for most people. However, some people should check with their doctor before they start becoming much more physically active.

If you are planning to become much more physically active than you are now, start by answering the seven questions in the box below. If you are between the ages of 15 and 69, the PAR-Q will tell you if you should check with your doctor before you start. If you are over 69 years of age, and you are not used to being very active, check with your doctor.

Common sense is your best guide when you answer these questions. Please read the questions carefully and answer each one honestly: check YES or NO.

YES	NO	
☐	☐	1. Has your doctor ever said that you have a heart condition <u>and</u> that you should only do physical activity recommended by a doctor?
☐	☐	2. Do you feel pain in your chest when you do physical activity?
☐	☐	3. In the past month, have you had chest pain when you were not doing physical activity?
☐	☐	4. Do you lose your balance because of dizziness or do you ever lose consciousness?
☐	☐	5. Do you have a bone or joint problem that could be made worse by a change in your physical activity?
☐	☐	6. Is your doctor currently prescribing drugs (for example, water pills) for your blood pressure or heart condition?
☐	☐	7. Do you know of <u>any other reason</u> why you should not do physical activity?

IF YOU ANSWERED

YES to one or more questions

Talk with your doctor by phone or in person BEFORE you start becoming much more physically active or BEFORE you have a fitness appraisal. Tell your doctor about the PAR-Q and which questions you answered YES.

- You may be able to do any activity you want—as long as you start slowly and build up gradually. Or, you may need to restrict your activities to those which are safe for you. Talk with your doctor about the kinds of activities you wish to participate in and follow his/her advice.
- Find out which community programs are safe and helpful for you.

NO to all questions

If you answered NO honestly to <u>all</u> PAR-Q questions, you can be reasonably sure that you can:

- start becoming much more physically active—begin slowly and build up gradually. This is the safest and easiest way to go.
- take part in a fitness appraisal—this is an excellent way to determine your basic fitness so that you can plan the best way for you to live actively.

DELAY BECOMING MUCH MORE ACTIVE:

- if you are not feeling well because of a temporary illness such as a cold or fever—wait until you feel better; or
- if you are or may be pregnant—talk to your doctor before you start becoming more active.

Please note: If your health changes so that you then answer YES to any of the above questions, tell your fitness or health professional. Ask whether you should change your physical activity plan.

you. Remember, if you're in doubt, err on the side of safety and check with your doctor.

SPECIAL ISSUES FOR WOMEN WITH OSTEOPOROSIS

If you have osteoporosis, speak with your doctor before starting this program.

Physical activity is particularly beneficial for women with low bone density—but it's important to observe certain precautions:

- Avoid exercises that require you to bend your back forward. However, it's safe to bend forward from the hip if you keep your back straight.
- Skip sports that involve high impact or risk of falling.
- If your coordination or balance is poor, use treadmills or stair climbers only if they have sturdy handrails.

The exercises in this book have been selected to be safe and beneficial for older women. Many of the moves have been used in research studies on older women, including participants with osteopenia or osteoporosis. Nevertheless, if you have osteoporosis, your particular needs may be different. Based on your condition and history, your doctor may advise you to adapt the program or to consult a physical therapist.

WEIGHT-BEARING AEROBIC ACTIVITY PROGRAM

If you aren't already doing weight-bearing aerobic exercise, this part of the *Strong Women, Strong Bones* program will help you get started. Once your body is strong and fit, it's a joy to be physically active. Many older women tell me that the combination of aerobic activity and strength training makes them feel twenty years younger.

Exercise options

Women often ask me, "What's the best aerobic activity for bones?" My answer is, we don't know yet. However, we believe that any weight-bearing activity is beneficial, provided it's done at sufficient intensity. A weight-bearing exercise is one that requires your legs to support most of your body weight—in other words, you're not seated or in the water. Thus your bones, especially your hip and spine bones, are stimulated.

I want to emphasize that occasional physical activity isn't what makes the difference with bone. Research shows that benefits come from *regular, repeated exercise*—from *habits* of physical activity. What's more, your body has to be well nourished to reap the rewards.

The easiest way to develop an exercise habit is to select an activity that's readily available and that you enjoy (or at least find tolerable). Of course, if you have osteoporosis or other concerns, the exercise must be safe and appropriate. I think it's helpful to have one "bread and butter" exercise—something you can count on doing three times a week, which easily becomes a routine part of your life. Some people, including me, love to get outdoors to exercise. They want to breathe fresh air; they want to go places and see the countryside. Others prefer indoor workouts, for equally valid reasons. They don't have to worry about the weather, traffic, or unsafe neighborhoods; or they like using exercise machines in front of the TV. Either way is fine.

If you're already doing weight-bearing aerobic exercise, you can continue (though you may want to do things a little differently after you've read this chapter). If you've been sedentary, I suggest you select one activity for the first few weeks. Once you become familiar with it, you can expand your repertoire. Variety prevents boredom; also, different activities stimulate different bones. Here are some possibilities:

Walking

Your leg and hip bones are stimulated every time your foot hits the ground. But because the stimulation is small, effects aren't visible for many years. However, walking provides the other benefits of aerobic exercise much more quickly.

Walking is an ideal aerobic activity for many women. It's simple and convenient, and easily tucked into your daily routine. Except during inclement weather when surfaces get slippery, walking is usually safe. Of course, women with osteoporosis need to avoid uneven ground so they don't fall.

The best way to adjust the intensity of your walking workout is to move faster or go uphill. Some women increase intensity by wearing ankle weights when they walk, but this is dangerous—especially if you have osteoporosis. Added weight can throw off your balance, which could lead to falls or joint problems.

If you prefer to walk on a treadmill, be aware that balance can be tricky, especially when you're a beginner. Keep a hand on the railings at first. But as soon as you're able, walk without holding on, because you'll have a better workout. To help maintain balance, find a focal point—something to look at that's straight ahead and about ten to twenty feet away. If you need to turn your head, don't just spin around; hold the handrail and turn slowly.

Jogging and running

Jogging and running have more impact on bone than walking. These are excellent activities for cardiovascular fitness as well. However, jogging and running can be hard on the joints, so they're risky for women with osteoporosis or other orthopedic problems.

Stair climbing

Several studies have shown that stair climbing increases the density of the hipbone. It's a terrific aerobic exercise, and also helps with coordination and balance. Even if you use another activity for your bread-and-butter exercise, I encourage you to take the stairs whenever you can. It's one of the easiest ways I've found to tuck extra aerobic exercise into my life. Stair climbing can be risky for individuals with osteoporosis or with balance or vision problems, so take special care. Also, stairs can elevate your heart rate very quickly. If you're heavy or very out of shape, you'll need to start slowly and progress gradually.

What about a stair-climbing machine? Like the real thing, this popular device provides great aerobic exercise. But you don't get the down portion of stair climbing, which is what creates the greatest impact on bone. So the benefits probably aren't the same as from real stairs.

Cross-country skiing, skating, elliptical walking machines

Skating and cross-country skiing provide great aerobic workouts. Their gliding movements are easy on the joints, which can be an important advantage. Unfortunately, these sports may not be safe if you have osteoporosis or balance problems. But most women can enjoy the machine version of cross-country skiing, as well as the similar motions of elliptical walkers. All of these activities are weight-bearing, but they don't create as much force on the skeleton as exercises in which your foot actually hits the ground. So for the best benefits to bone, higher-impact exercise is needed as well.

Aerobics classes

Classes—the options range from boxing to tap dancing—provide an enjoyable weight-bearing aerobic workout. Most improve coordination and balance. Instructors usually include a warm-up, cool-down, and stretch. Before you select a class, read a description or talk with the instructor to find out if the required fitness level is appropriate for you. If you have balance problems or osteoporosis, choose a class that won't put you at risk for falling.

Exercise videos let you bring some of the fun of an aerobics class into your home. If possible, rent a video before you buy, to make sure it's appropriate and enjoyable.

Rowing

Though rowing isn't a weight-bearing exercise, it generates considerable force on the hips and back. Because of this, rowing is not advised for women with osteoporosis. However, it can be an excellent option for those with joint problems that make weight-bearing exercise difficult. One study of an exercise program that combined rowing with strength training found improvements in bone density at the hip and spine.

Tennis and other racket sports

Research shows that women who regularly play tennis and other racket sports have denser bones than sedentary women, especially in the playing arm. These activities also promote aerobic fitness. And since they require agility and coordination, they train balance too.

If you have the partners and facilities to enjoy racket sports regularly, they're a great bread-and-butter activity. However, they're not advisable for women with balance problems or osteoporosis because of the risk of falling. If you're a beginner, get in shape before you start—otherwise it's easy to injure yourself.

Team sports

Active team sports—like basketball, soccer, volleyball, and field hockey—can provide excellent weight-bearing exercise and balance training, plus the motivational power of regularly scheduled sessions and workout partners. Like racket sports, team sports are risky for women with balance problems or osteoporosis. And it's important to get in shape before you start, to avoid injuries.

General instructions for weight-bearing aerobic workouts

Here are a few suggestions to make your workouts safer, more effective, and more enjoyable.

Dress for success

Some women get a boost from stylish exercise gear, but if you prefer to keep it simple, a loose cotton T-shirt plus shorts or leggings are just fine.

- Select shoes that fit well. Good athletic shoes can be expensive, but they're worth it because they help prevent injuries and discomfort. Weight-bearing activity is hard on shoes—and worn-out shoes are hard on your body. Examine footwear at least once a month, and replace or repair it promptly if needed.
- Wear layers that you can peel off as your body warms up.
- Use all recommended safety gear, such as reflecting strips on clothing if you walk at night.

Check the equipment

If you're using equipment—whether it's a tennis racket or a treadmill—give it a quick look-over before each workout to make sure it's in good repair. Follow all maintenance suggestions in the manual.

Drink plenty of water

Your body requires extra water when you're active. To stay well hydrated, drink at least one cup of water during the hour before an aerobic workout. Then drink another cup or two within the forty-five minutes following aerobic activity. If an activity is prolonged—for instance, if you're taking a long hike—drink half a cup of water every fifteen minutes or so. You need even more water on hot days, when your body has to work harder to stay cool.

Warm up

Muscles work best when they're warm: they're more elastic and have a better supply of blood. So it's important to warm your muscles before you place heavy demands on them. This is especially true for older people and those with cardiovascular disease.

A warm-up need not be elaborate or take extra time. Simply begin your exercise at a slow, easy pace, rather than at full speed. Take five minutes to reach your target intensity. This gradual transition from a resting to an active state gives your body time to adjust.

Cool down and stretch

The cool-down is just as simple as the warm-up, only in reverse: Over a five-minute period, slow your pace. After you're finished you can do your strengthening exercises if you're combining the two into a single workout session.

End every exercise session with a stretch. Stretching is particularly important after an aerobic workout because most aerobic activities work your muscles at high intensity, but through only a limited range of motion. If you don't stretch afterwards, you can actually decrease your flexibility. The three simple stretches described on pages 206–13 prevent that problem—and they feel great!

How to gauge aerobic effort

The key to getting results from aerobic exercise is to work out at the right intensity. In this program, your heart will work at about 60 to 80 percent of its maximum most of the time. This is safely within your capability, but high enough to give your cardiovascular system a good workout. How do you know you're at the right level? In the laboratory, we use heart rate–monitoring equipment and a 20-point exercise-intensity scale to measure aerobic effort. But you can refer to the simpler intensity scale below or check your pulse.

Estimating exercise intensity

The easiest way to measure your effort is with a subjective scale that describes how you're feeling as you exercise. You can use the scale at any point in your workout, and you don't need special apparatus. Though this system generally works well, I encourage you also to take your pulse a few times at the beginning (I'll tell you how in a minute), to make sure your impressions match your actual heart rate.

EXERCISE INTENSITY SCALE FOR WEIGHT-BEARING ACTIVITY	
EXERCISE INTENSITY LEVEL	DESCRIPTION OF EFFORT
1—Sedentary	No perceived effort; standing, sitting, or lying down.
2—Active This level contributes to overall health and burns more calories than being sedentary.	Easy, sustainable movement that causes a small increase in heart and breathing rate and doesn't raise a sweat (unless the weather is hot), such as strolling, gardening, slow dancing, golfing.
3—Aerobic training Exercise at this level conditions your heart and lungs.	Somewhat hard movement that elevates the heart rate to 60 to 70 percent of maximum most of the time, ranging up to 80 percent. Breathing is more rapid, though it's possible to converse with only slightly altered speech; perspiration appears after about five to fifteen minutes, depending on air temperature.
4—Athletic training This is a more advanced level of aerobic conditioning that might become an appropriate goal after the twelve-week program.	Hard effort that elevates the heart rate to 70 to 80 percent most of the time, ranging up to 90 percent of maximum. Breathing is more rapid but not labored—it's possible to converse, though faster breathing will cause evident interruptions; perspiration will start within five to ten minutes depending on air temperature; fatigue will increase as the workout continues and you will feel a need to stop by the end.
5—Overexertion Not recommended!	Excessive effort: heart pounds to the point of discomfort or nausea; breathing is too rapid to permit speech.

The *Strong Women, Strong Bones* weight-bearing aerobic exercise program calls for level 3 effort at least three times a week. But I hope you'll also make level 2 activity part of your daily life as you become stronger and fitter. The more active you are, the more stimulation your bones will receive—and the more calories you'll burn.

Measuring your heart rate

Heart rate monitors can be purchased at sporting goods stores, but the good ones are expensive ($60 and up). Fortunately you can get the same information by taking your pulse. All you need is a clock or watch with a second hand—and a little practice. Here's how:

- Hold your right hand out. Press the forefinger and middle finger of your left hand together and touch them to the base of your right thumb. Slide the fingers across your wrist, moving them parallel to the top of your right arm. You'll feel a narrow hollow in your right forearm between the bone on top and the tendons below. Press firmly when you're at the hollow. You should be able to feel your pulse. It may help to bend your right wrist back slightly.
- Watching the clock, count the number of beats you feel for fifteen seconds. Multiply the number by 4 to get your heart rate (beats per minute).

Check your heart rate when you're five minutes into aerobic activity, or at the end before you cool down. And of course, you can check it whenever you want to know how hard you're working. Two cautions:

- Don't take your pulse at your neck, by pressing on your carotid artery—that could impede blood flow to your brain.
- If you're using a pacemaker or taking medications that can raise or lower your heart rate—including cold remedies, appetite suppressants, or calcium channel blockers for blood pressure—discuss exercise-intensity goals with your doctor before you start.

Target heart rate for aerobic exercise

To be effective, an aerobic workout should raise your heart rate. Your **target heart rate** for exercise is 60 to 80 percent of your **maximum heart rate.** Your maximum heart rate decreases with age. Use the table to determine your target heart rate.

TARGET HEART RATE

MAXIMUM HEART RATE = 220 minus your age in years

TARGET HEART RATE = 60 to 80 percent of MAXIMUM HEART RATE

	HEART RATE IN BEATS PER MINUTE AT DIFFERENT PERCENTS OF MAXIMUM			
AGE	60%	70%	80%	90%
20	120	140	160	180
25	117	137	156	176
30	114	133	152	171
35	111	130	148	167
40	108	126	144	162
45	105	123	140	158
50	102	119	136	153
55	99	116	132	149
60	96	112	128	144
65	93	109	124	140
70	90	105	120	135
75	87	102	116	131
80	84	98	112	126

Creating an individualized weight-bearing aerobic exercise program

If you're already doing weight-bearing aerobic exercise, don't stop! You might want to adjust your workouts to be sure the intensity level is appropriate.

If you're new to aerobic exercise, begin gradually and progress steadily as described below. You'll be surprised by how painlessly you can transform yourself from sedentary to fit.

WEEKLY PROGRESS GOALS

Minutes of level 3 weight-bearing aerobic activity

WEEK	MINUTES PER SESSION	DAYS PER WEEK
1	15	3
2	15	3
3	15	3
4	20	3
5	20	3
6	20	3
7	20	3
8	25	3
9	25	3
10	25	3
11	25	3
12	30	3

I'm frequently asked if it's okay to split aerobic exercise into two sessions a day. Yes, it is—two fifteen-minute workouts are just as good as a single thirty-minute workout. Remember that you still need to warm up and cool down for each mini-session.

After twelve weeks you can stick with three thirty-minute exercise sessions per week. Or you can increase the length of your workouts or the number of days you exercise. To avoid injuries and muscle soreness, advance slowly: each week add no more than one day of exercise or five minutes per workout. For instance, in week 13 you could do three thirty-five-minute workouts or four thirty-minute workouts.

Be sure to take at least one day of rest every week. Studies find that people who overdo aerobic exercise by training seven days a week have more injuries than those who take a weekly break.

HIGH-IMPACT EXERCISE PROGRAM

An exciting new exercise with proven bone benefits is vertical jumping. Just two minutes per day of vertical jumping can produce significant improvements in the hipbones in a matter of months. This is the single most efficient form of exercise for the bones. Unfortunately, vertical jumping is not for everyone. Only premenopausal women who don't have osteoporosis can safely benefit from this form of exercise.

Before you start

Vertical jumping builds bone because it's a high-impact activity. For the very same reason, vertical jumping is hard on joints and risky for individuals with established osteoporosis. If you're premenopausal and already fit, you can begin vertical jumping now. Otherwise, wait until after the first twelve weeks to start jumping.

IMPORTANT: Skip high-impact exercise if you're postmenopausal, if you have osteoporosis or compromised balance, or if you have a history of knee, ankle, or back problems.

General instructions

Perform the vertical jumps after you've finished your weight-bearing aerobic activity—that way your body will be warmed up. On days when you aren't doing an aerobic workout, warm up by walking for five minutes before jumping.

ABOUT THE SCIENCE

Getting the jump on osteoporosis

Dr. Joan Bassey of the Queen's Medical Centre in Nottingham, England, has demonstrated 2 to 5 percent increases in hipbone density in women who performed a simple two-minute exercise routine daily for six months. These results are among the best that have ever been reported in a scientific study about exercise for bone.

The subjects were twenty-seven women in their twenties and thirties who attended a weekly low-impact exercise class at a community center. During the study, fourteen of the women substituted fifty vertical jumps for some of the class exercises; they also did fifty vertical jumps every day at home. The control group continued their usual workout in class and did a low-intensity arm exercise at home. The result after just six months: significant increases in hipbone density from vertical jumping.

You can jump on nearly any flat surface, indoors or out. Just avoid slippery spots or extremely hard surfaces such as concrete, ceramic tile, or metal. Wood and firm ground are fine. Wear shoes to protect your feet.

Begin each session with a few warm-up jumps at less than maximal effort. These warm-ups don't count toward your total.

THE EXERCISES

Start with the jumping jack. After four weeks, you can progress to the power jump—provided that you can easily do the jumping jack in good form and your joints don't hurt.

JUMPING JACK ◆

This exercise is a modified version of the traditional jumping jack. It's appropriate for fit, healthy premenopausal women with good balance.

Starting position: Stand with your feet together and your arms at your sides, palms facing in.

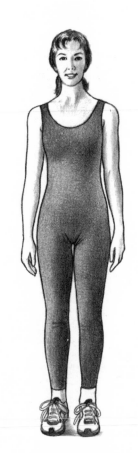

Jump out: Bend your knees *slightly* and then jump. Simultaneously move your arms and feet directly out to the sides. Your feet should be approximately 3 feet apart. Your arms should be parallel to the floor. Land on the balls of your feet with your knees slightly bent.

Pause for a moment.

Jump in: Jump and return your feet and arms to the starting position, landing on the balls of your feet with slightly bent knees.

Pause for a breath, then repeat the move.

Reps: Perform a total of 10 jumps to begin with. Each week, add another 5 jumps. Work up to 50 jumps. Do these jumps three to six days per week.

Notes from your personal trainer:

You'll feel the effort in your feet, lower legs, and thighs—the entire leg. If you feel the effort in your knees, make sure they aren't locked. No matter how small the jump, your knees should be slightly bent when you land.

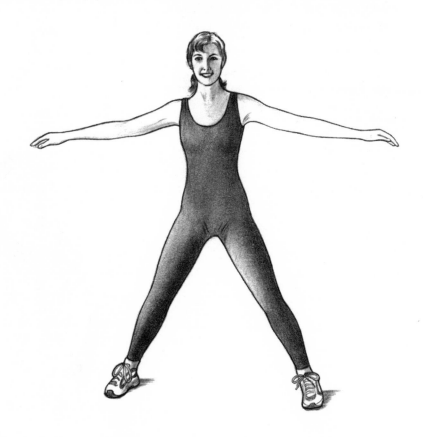

POWER JUMP ◆

This exercise is a modified version of an athletic move called the vertical jump. Advance to this exercise only after you have performed the jumping jack for at least four weeks and are certain you can jump and land safely.

Starting position: Stand with your feet hip-width apart and your elbows bent slightly, palms facing in. Focus your eyes slightly upward to anticipate the upward movement of the jump.

Jump up: Bend your knees 4 to 6 inches, then jump straight up. The height of your jump will depend upon your leg strength. As you jump, extend your arms up over your head, as if you were reaching toward the ceiling. Land on the balls of your feet with slightly bent knees.

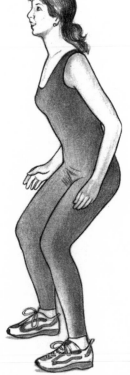

Pause for a breath, then repeat the move.

Reps: Perform a total of 10 jumps to begin with. Each week add 5 jumps, working up to a total of 50 jumps. Do these jumps three to six days a week.

Notes from your personal trainer:

You'll feel the effort in your feet, lower legs, and thighs—the entire leg. If you feel the effort in your knees, make sure they aren't locked. No matter how small the jump, your knees should be slightly bent when you land.

As you become more comfortable with the jump, challenge yourself by trying to jump higher.

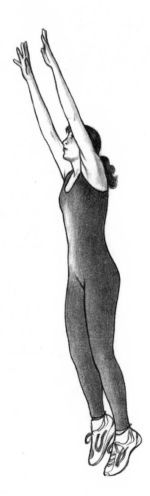

Jumping rope

We don't yet have research quantifying the bone benefits of jumping rope, but it's an excellent aerobic exercise that stimulates your heart, muscles, and skeleton. Since you're not jumping as high as you do with vertical jumping, it may not be as effective for building bone, so I don't recommend it as your only high-impact activity. But by all means, include jumping rope in your weight-bearing aerobic exercise if you enjoy it.

Jumping rope is a challenging, high-impact activity. If you have knee, back, hip, or other joint problems, it's not for you. It's best to be in good shape before you begin. Here are some tips:

- **The gear:** Get a jump rope with handles that is thick and heavy enough to swing well. Check the length by stepping on the rope with one foot—the handles should just reach your arm pits. Wear sturdy shoes—sneakers are fine.
- **The preliminaries:** Because you can't start jumping rope slowly, warm up with another aerobic activity for five minutes.
- **The workout:** Start by jumping for just one minute; rest for thirty seconds; then jump for another minute. Limit your first session to five cycles—a total of five minutes of jumping. After you finish, cool down and stretch—this is very important for avoiding injuries.
- **To progress:** Wait a day or two to see how you feel. You may experience delayed muscle soreness in your calves and ankles. Slowly build your workout, each week adding thirty seconds of jumping to each cycle. For instance, in the second week, instead of jumping for a minute in each cycle, you can jump for a minute and a half. Advance slowly until you can jump without breaks for as long as you like.
- **Cautions:** Pay attention to your body as you jump. If you're working so hard that you can barely talk, it's too strenuous. (See the intensity scale for aerobic exercise on page 146.)

STRENGTH-TRAINING PROGRAM

I've worked with women of all ages, fitness levels, and body types. Though many of them are skeptical about strength training at first, nearly everyone loves it once they get started. Their body shape becomes more youthful and they have more strength and energy; becoming strong makes them feel empowered physically and emotionally. Knowing that these exercises build stronger bones is a further motivation.

A special note for readers of my first two books: If you're already following the strength-training program in *Strong Women Stay Young* or *Strong Women Stay Slim,* you can continue—or you can switch to the strengthening exercises in this book, which focus on bone benefits. The box on pages 197–98 offers recommendations.

Gear

To strengthen your muscles, you must work them harder than usual. That's why several of the exercises use dumbbells and ankle weights. Most of the necessary equipment can be found at discount and department stores, but you might need to visit a sporting goods store. See the resource box on page 158 for mail order and online sources. Here's what you need:

Dumbbells
For the first few weeks, you'll use two pairs of dumbbells: a 3-pound pair and a 5-pound pair. Later, as you become stronger, you'll need pairs of 6-, 8-, and 10-pound dumbbells; some women will need 12- and 15-pounders. Expect to pay about $5 each for the 3-pound weights and $7 each for the 5-pounders. Heavier weights cost a little more.

Ankle weights
Starting with week 8, you'll need ankle weights—strap-on cuffs with compartments that hold weighted bars. You adjust the weight of the cuff by adding or removing these bars.

- If you're age 50 or younger, or age 50 to 70 and physically fit, buy two 20-pound cuffs.

- If you're age 70 or older, or age 50 to 70 and out of shape, buy two 10-pound cuffs.

Ten-pound ankle weights cost about $30 each; 20-pound cuffs cost around $50 each. Note: You can buy just one cuff; however, the routine will take longer if you have to switch it from leg to leg.

Strength-training equipment sources

All Pro Exercise Products, Inc.
PO Box 8268
Longboat Key, FL 34228
800/735-9287
fax: 941/387-7901
http://www.allproweights.com

Keiser Sports Health Equipment
2470 South Cherry Avenue
Fresno, CA 93706
800/888-7009; 559/256-8000
fax: 559/256-8100

Fitness Distributors
17 South Avenue
Natick, MA 01760
800/244-1882; 508/653-1882
fax: 508/650-0448

Country Technology, Inc.
PO Box 87
Gays Mills, WI 54631
608/735-4718
fax: 608/735-4859

MC Sports
3070 Shaffer Street, S.E.
Grand Rapids, MI 49512
800/626-1762; 616/942-2600
fax: 616/942-1973

Paragon Sporting Goods
871 Broadway
New York, NY 10003
212/255-8036
fax: 212/929-1831

Fitness First
PO Box 251
Shawnee Mission, KS 66201
800/421-1791; 913/384-6262
fax: 800/421-0036
http://www.fitness1st.com

Intellbell's PowerBlock
1819 South Cedar Avenue
Owatonna, MN 55060
800/446-5215
http://www.powerblock.com

Chair

You'll do some of the exercises while seated in a chair. Select a sturdy chair without arms. Often a dining room chair is just right.

Staircase or step

One exercise requires a staircase or an exercise step. If you don't have access to a staircase with a hand railing, you can purchase a step. Exercise steps are available at sporting goods stores, but they can be expensive ($30 to $100). A less expensive alternative ($10 to $20) is a sturdy utility step 8 to 12 inches tall; these are sold at hardware stores. Make sure that the step has four solid legs and a skid-proof top, and that it can hold your body weight easily without tipping over.

Exercise mat (optional)

A firm exercise mat makes floor exercises more comfortable. Or you can use a large bath towel. Place the towel or mat on a rug, if possible, for added cushioning.

Towel

One of the cool-down stretches requires a towel. The same towel can be put under your head for the floor exercises.

What to wear

You don't need special clothing for strength training. However, I recommend the following for comfort:

- Thick socks or leg warmers to prevent the ankle weights from chafing
- Sturdy, supportive shoes—such as sneakers or athletic shoes—that have a sole flexible enough for you to stand on your toes

General instructions for strength training

Strength training is safe for nearly everyone. But it's important to heed the simple precautions below, which also make for more effective workouts.

Create a safe exercise area

Clear a space for training. Stow weights in a sturdy box or other secure location when you're not using them, and keep them safely away from children and pets.

Back safety tips

Caution: If you've ever had back problems, or if you have established osteoporosis, discuss this program with your doctor before you begin.

The following tips are for everyone—but pay special attention if you need to pamper your back.

- Be just as careful when moving weights to and from the workout area as you are when you do the exercises. If possible, store your dumbbells next to your workout area, so you don't have to move them for each session.
- When you pick up the weights, do it properly. Bend at the legs and rise slowly. Do not bend forward as you lift—that puts pressure on the spine, which can cause fractures.

Maintain good posture

Proper posture helps you avoid muscle strain and injury. As you grow stronger, good posture becomes easier. If you already have curvature of the spine from osteoporosis, strengthening your back muscles will help you stand as tall as possible—and will also reduce pain and fatigue.

Count out loud while you exercise

If you count, you automatically breathe properly—inhaling before you start the move, and exhaling as you lift and lower the weight. Counting aloud also reminds you to move slowly, which makes the moves safer and more effective.

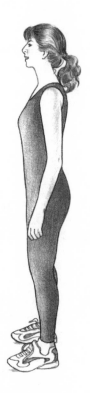

Good posture

Whether you're sitting or standing, your body should be relaxed but straight, as if someone had fastened a string to the top of your head and was pulling you up. Check yourself in a mirror:

- *Chin is tipped in, so it's in line with your neck.*
- *Neck is in line with your spine.*
- *Shoulders are slightly drawn back, down, and relaxed.*
- *Back is straight.*
- *Pelvis is slightly tucked under.*
- *Knees are neither locked nor bent.*

Progress at the recommended pace

Some women become so enthusiastic about strength training that they press forward too quickly and hurt themselves. It's important to allow your muscles at least a day of rest between workouts. Don't exercise the same muscle two days in a row.

Relax!

Don't hold your breath as you lift the weights—a common mistake. Breathing properly helps you relax.

As you do the exercises, check your body for tension:

- **Face:** Keep your face relaxed; don't furrow or knit your brow.

- **Jaw and neck:** Avoid clenching your teeth or tightening your jaw. If your jaw is relaxed, your neck will be relaxed too.

- **Shoulders:** Don't scrunch your shoulders up toward your ears. Keep them back and relaxed.

- **Legs and arms:** Only the muscles you're exercising should be tensed. All other muscles in your body should be relaxed. Don't lock your knees.

How to do the exercises

In strength training, a complete move is called a **lift** or a **repetition** or **rep.** In this program, eight reps make a **set,** and you do two sets of each exercise.

A lift takes about nine seconds: four seconds to raise the weight, a one-second pause, and four seconds to return to the starting position. You'll stop for a few seconds to take a breath between lifts. Rest about one minute between sets. Though it's not necessary, you may want to pause for a minute or two when you finish an exercise before you go on to the next.

The key to strength training is to begin slowly and progress consistently. You'll start with light weights or the easiest version of the exercise. At first you'll progress rapidly, and within a few weeks you'll be training at the proper intensity: You'll be able to perform each exercise eight times in good form, but this effort should be close to your limit. When the eighth lift is no longer a challenge, it's time to increase the load.

WEEKS 1 TO 3

Begin with these four exercises. You'll use dumbbells for some of them.

EXERCISE 1: WIDE LEG SQUAT ♦

All you need is a chair to do this wonderfully practical exercise. In a single move, you'll strengthen the muscles of your front, back, and inner thigh as well as your buttocks. That makes it especially helpful for the hipbones. At the same time, the exercise requires balance and spatial awareness—which help prevent falls. What's more, the exercise serves as a warm-up, which makes your workout more efficient.

Starting position: Place the chair on a rug or against a wall so it doesn't slide. Stand about 6 inches in front of the chair with your feet a little wider than shoulder-width apart and your toes turned slightly outward. Cross your arms in front of your chest. Keep your shoulders relaxed and your eyes focused straight ahead. Lean forward slightly from the hip, with your chest lifted and your back, neck, and head in a straight line.

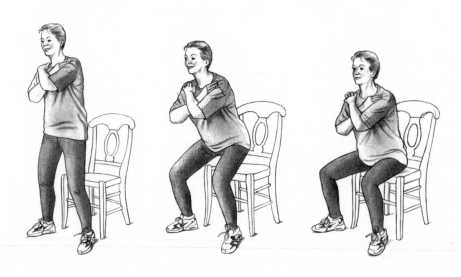

1-2-3-Down: Take a deep breath, then aim your buttocks back and slowly lower yourself into the chair. Your knees should remain above your ankles; they don't move forward.

Pause for a moment in the seated position.

1-2-3-Up: Lean forward slightly and slowly stand. Your knees should remain above your ankles. Push up from your heels through your lower leg, thigh, hips, and buttocks until you're standing up straight.

Pause for a breath, then repeat the move.

Reps and sets: Repeat until you have done 8 chair squats—this is 1 set. Rest for a minute or two and do a second set.

Notes from your personal trainer:

Make sure your chest remains lifted throughout the move, so your body doesn't curl forward. Focus your eyes on a spot in front of you rather than looking down—that will help. You'll feel the effort in the front and back of your thighs, your buttocks, and your lower back. If this move hurts your knees, you're probably making the common mistake of letting them move forward as you squat. Concentrate on keeping your knees above your ankles. Your lower leg should remain perpendicular to the floor.

If the move is too difficult, try lowering yourself just a few inches or put a thick pillow on the chair to make it easier. As you get stronger, you can advance.

When you're ready for more, try these variations:

- Lower your body almost to the chair, but don't sit. Hold yourself in position for a breath, and then rise.
- Hold one dumbbell in each hand, cross your hands over your chest, and do the exercise with the added weight.

EXERCISE 2: STEP UP ◆

You'll strengthen the muscles on the front and back of the thigh with this challenging exercise, so you'll strengthen your hipbones. This move also improves balance and coordination.

Starting position: Stand close to the bottom step of a sturdy staircase that has a hand railing. Hold the railing lightly for support. Step up to the first step with one leg, placing your foot squarely on the first step, toes pointing forward. Your torso should be upright with your head up and eyes focused straight ahead. Make sure the knee of your front leg is directly over your ankle and does not move past your toes.

1-2-3-Up: Lift your body straight up with the muscles of your front leg so that your back foot reaches the level of the first step. Tap the toes of your back foot on the step while keeping your body weight supported by your front leg.

Pause for a breath.

1-2-3-Down: Slowly return to the starting position. Concentrate on supporting your body weight with the front leg as you move down.

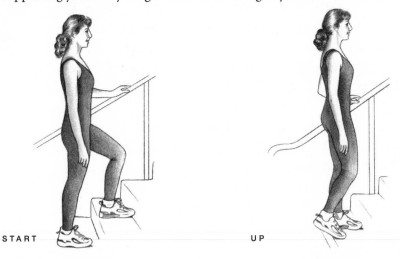

START   UP

Pause for a breath, and then repeat the move with the same front leg. Your foot should remain on the first step while you complete all reps in the set.

Reps and sets: Repeat until you have done 8 reps with the same leg; then perform 8 reps with the other leg—that is 1 set. Rest for a minute or two and do a second set.

Notes from your personal trainer:

You will feel the effort in the front and back of the forward thigh. If you don't feel the effort in that leg, you're probably pushing off with your back leg rather than pulling up with the front leg.

If you feel discomfort in your front knee, you may be letting your knee come forward over your toe. Concentrate on keeping your knee over your ankle as you move up and down.

When you're ready to progress, start with your front foot on the second step instead of the first. After that you can add challenge by holding a dumbbell in each hand and keeping your arms crossed over your chest as you do the move. Start with 3-pound dumbbells and slowly progress as you get stronger.

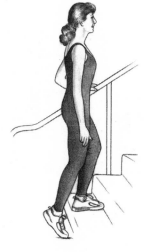

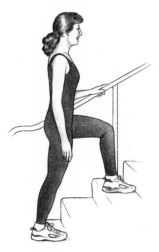

DOWN   TWO-STEP VERSION

EXERCISE 3: SEATED OVERHEAD PRESS ◆

The muscles and bones of the upper spine and shoulder are strengthened by this exercise. One result is improved posture—an important benefit for women with osteoporosis in the spine.

Starting position: Sit upright toward the front of the chair with your feet flat on the floor about hip-width apart. Hold one dumbbell in each hand. Keeping your upper arms to the sides of your body, bend your elbows to bring your forearms all the way up. The weights should be at shoulder height parallel to the floor, with the inner ends just in front of your shoulders. Your palms should face forward and your wrists should be straight.

1-2-3 -Up: Slowly press the dumbbells straight up. Extend your arms, but don't lock your elbows. The weights will be just in front of your head, not directly above it.

Pause for a breath.

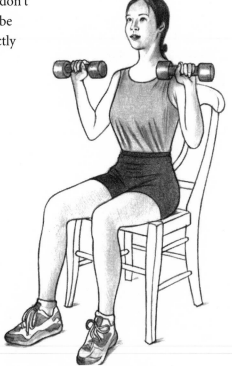

1-2-3-Down: Slowly return to the starting position.

Pause for a breath, and then repeat the move.

Reps and sets: Repeat for 8 reps—this is 1 set. Rest and repeat a second set of 8 reps.

Notes from your personal trainer:

You'll feel the effort in your shoulders, arms, and upper back. Don't lean back. Maintain good posture during the move; don't scrunch your shoulders or arch your back. Keep your wrists straight—don't let them bend backward as you do the move.

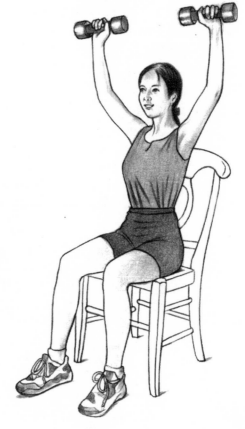

EXERCISE 4: FORWARD FLY ♦

When you strengthen the muscles of your shoulders and upper back, the bones get stronger too. This exercise also improves posture. If you already have some curvature of the spine, strengthening your upper-back muscles will help you correct your posture as much as possible. Caution: If you have crush fractures or curvature of the spine, be sure to discuss this exercise with your doctor. Because you're bending from the hips, the exercise is safe for nearly everyone.

Starting position: Sit in the chair with your feet flat on the floor, hip-width apart. Your thigh and lower leg should be perpendicular to each other. Holding a dumbbell in each hand, bend forward from your *hips* approximately 3 to 5 inches. Your back should be flat and your spine straight—the forward movement comes from your hips. Hold the dumbbells straight up in front of your chest with your palms facing in. Bend your elbows slightly, as if you were hugging a tree.

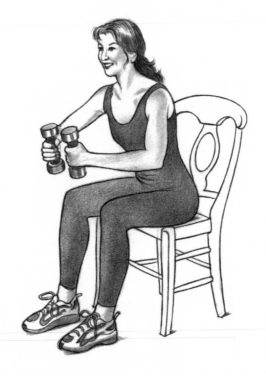

1-2-3-Back: Pull your shoulder blades together, moving your elbows as far back as possible. Keep your arms slightly bent throughout the move.

Pause for a moment.

1-2-3-Forward: Slowly bring your arms back to the starting position.

Pause for a breath, then repeat the move.

Reps and sets: Repeat until you have done 8 reps—this is 1 set. Rest for a minute or two and do a second set.

Notes from your personal trainer:

You will feel the effort in your shoulders, upper back, and arms. The movement should originate in your shoulder blades. Focus on moving the shoulder muscles rather than moving your arms. Elbows remain bent at the same angle throughout the move. Be careful not to arch or move your back.

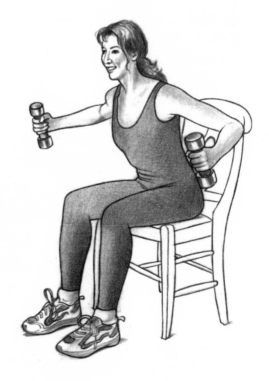

Optional Extra: Wrist Curl

Clinical research trials have shown that this simple move increases bone density in the wrist. If you have weak wrists—or if you're concerned about osteoporosis in your wrists—I encourage you to do this exercise.

Caution: If you've already had a wrist fracture, talk with your physical therapist or physician first to make sure the move is safe for you.

Starting position: Sit all the way back in a chair with your thighs slightly separated, feet flat on the floor. Hold a dumbbell in each hand, palms facing down. Keeping your back straight, lean forward from the hips and rest your forearms on your thighs. Your wrist should extend past your knees.

1-2-3-Up: Lift both hands up and back toward your body. Your forearm should remain supported on your thigh.

Pause for a breath.

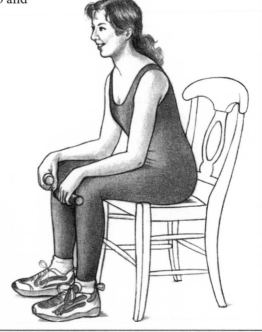

1-2-3-Down: Slowly lower your hands back to the starting position. Be sure that your back remains straight throughout the move.

Pause for a breath, then repeat the move.

Reps and sets: Repeat the move 8 times—1 set. Rest and do a second set.

Notes from your personal trainer:

You'll feel the effort in your forearm and wrist. This is a challenging exercise, so start with 1-pound weights. Or do the move with no weight at first, then gradually build up. If it's too difficult to place your forearms on your thighs, rest your arms on a table instead.

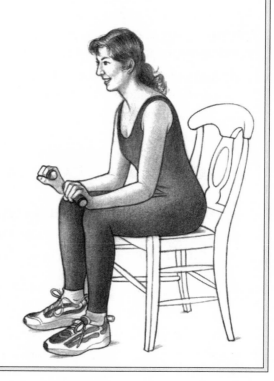

WEEKS 4 TO 7

Add the following two exercises to the four you've been doing. These are the first of several exercises done on the floor. If you don't ordinarily get up and down from the floor, please use sensible cautions:

- If you aren't certain that it's safe for you to do floor exercises, talk to your doctor first.
- If getting up and down is a struggle, do the exercises when someone is available to help you. Or wait an extra month to give yourself time to get stronger.

Here's one way to get up and down safely:

To go down: Position a sturdy chair on a rug or against a wall so it won't slip. Place one hand on the seat of the chair. Go down onto one knee; then go down onto the other knee. Take your hand off the chair and put it on the floor for support. Lie down on your side. Depending on the starting position for the exercise, roll onto your back or your front.

To get up: Roll onto your side. Using your hands for support, get onto your knees. Put a hand on the chair to steady yourself. Move one knee forward and up, and place the foot flat on the floor. Rise to a standing position.

EXERCISE 5: BACK EXTENSION ◆

This exercise strengthens the muscles in your buttocks as well as the back muscles that support your spine. Strengthening these muscles stimulates the bones of your hip and spine.

Starting position: Lie facedown on a mat or towel with your legs straight and toes pointed so that the laces of your sneakers face the floor. Place your right arm down along your side and place your left arm straight up above your head. Your right palm should face up, while your left palm faces down.

1-2-3-Up: Raise your right leg and left arm as high off the floor as you comfortably can. Lift your leg from the hip, keeping it straight. As you lift your arm, your head and neck will rise too; they should stay in line with the arm. Try to move your arm and leg simultaneously and as smoothly as possible.

Pause for a breath in the lifted position.

1-2-3-Down: Slowly return to the starting position.

Pause for a breath, then repeat the move. Complete 1 set and then raise your right arm, chest, and left leg.

Reps and sets: Repeat until you have done 8 reps with the same leg and opposite arm; then alternate and perform 8 reps with the other leg and arm—this is 1 set. Rest for a minute or two and do a second set.

Notes from your personal trainer:

You should feel the effort in your buttocks and in your entire back. Keep your nose pointed to the floor to make sure your head remains in proper alignment with your back. As your back muscles become stronger, you'll be able to lift your leg and arm higher off the floor. When you're ready for a more challenging workout, raise not only your arm but also your shoulder and upper chest as you lift your leg.

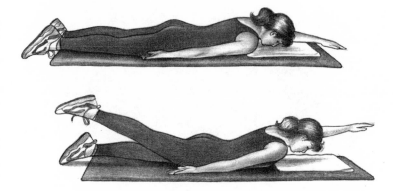

EXERCISE 6A: ABDOMINAL EXERCISE 1— Tummy Tuck ◆

Strengthening your abdominal muscles is one of the best things you can do for good posture. The combination of strong muscles in your back and abdomen helps stabilize your torso and protect your spine. Of course, tighter abs look better too.

Use the first version of the exercise until it's no longer challenging. Then move up to the second version, which is more difficult.

Starting position: Lie on your back with your knees bent and your feet flat on the floor. Your feet should be hip-width apart and approximately 12 to 18 inches from your buttocks. Place one hand on your stomach so you can feel your abdominal muscles working as you do the move. Your other arm should be extended straight at your side with the palm facing down.

1-2-3-Up: Press the small of your back against the floor and contract your abdominal muscles, tilting your pelvis toward your shoulders. Your pelvis and the bottom of your buttocks should come up only a few inches off the floor.

Pause for a breath.

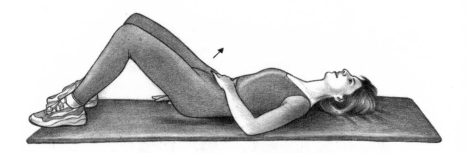

1-2-3-Down: Slowly return to the starting position.

Pause for a breath, then repeat the move.

Reps and sets: Repeat until you have done 8 tummy tuck moves—this is 1 set. Rest for a minute or two and do a second set.

Notes from your personal trainer:

Keep the small of your back pressed to the floor throughout the exercise. You should be able to feel your abdominal muscles contract with the hand that is resting on your stomach. If you feel the effort in front of your thighs, that means you're using your leg muscles instead of your abdominal muscles. Focus on keeping your thighs relaxed, and concentrate on tilting rather than lifting. At first you may move only a small distance. As you get stronger, you'll be able to lift your hips a little higher by just contracting your abdominal muscles.

EXERCISE 6B: ABDOMINAL EXERCISE 2— Reverse Curl ◆

When the tummy tuck is no longer challenging—and you're easily able to bring your entire buttocks off the floor in a steady movement—substitute the reverse curl. This is a more difficult move that also strengthens your abdominal muscles.

Starting position: Lie on your back with your knees bent, thighs together, and the small of your back pressed against the floor. Lift your feet off the floor approximately 5 to 8 inches so that your thighs are perpendicular to your body. Place one hand on your stomach so you can feel your abdominal muscles working when you do the move. Extend the other arm straight at your side with the palm facing down.

1-2-3-Up: Contract your abdominal muscles to lift the bottom of your buttocks up and back toward your shoulders. Your knees will move approximately 1 to 3 inches as you lift, coming up slightly and toward your chest.

Pause for a breath.

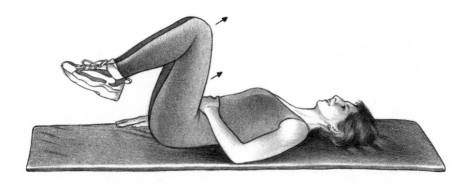

1-2-3-Down: Slowly move your buttocks and thighs back to the starting position.

Pause for a breath, then repeat. The small of your back should remain on the mat while you complete all reps in the set.

Reps and sets: Repeat until you have done 8 reverse curls—this is 1 set. Rest for a minute or two and do a second set.

Notes from your personal trainer:

Remember to exhale as you do the moves! A common mistake with this exercise is to hold your breath.

You should be able to feel your muscles contract with the hand that's resting on your stomach. If you feel the effort in your lower back, that means you're not keeping it pressed against the mat during the move. If your knees bend all the way to your chest, you're probably rocking your lower body and using your hip muscles instead of your abdominal muscles, which means you're not getting the benefit of this move. If this exercise is too difficult, return to the tummy tuck until you're stronger.

WEEKS 8 TO 11

Add two more exercises, bringing the total to eight. You will need ankle weights for these moves.

EXERCISE 7: SIDE LEG RAISE ◆

This is one of the best exercises for strengthening the muscles and bones of the hip and thigh. Developing the muscles on the outside of your hip is also important for agility and balance.

Starting position: Strap an ankle weight on each leg. Lie on the floor on your left side with your legs straight and together, one on top of the other. Bend the lower part of your left leg back behind you, making sure to keep your hips and knees aligned. Support your head with your left arm and place your right hand on the floor in front of you for balance.

1-2-3-Up: In a slow, controlled movement, lift your top leg while still keeping your trunk straight. The lifted leg should be straight, with the foot flat and toes pointed straight ahead.

Pause for a breath.

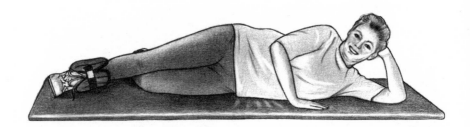

1-2-3-Down: Slowly return to the starting position.

Pause for a breath, and then repeat the move with the same leg.

Reps and sets: Repeat until you've competed 8 reps. Then roll onto your other side and do 8 reps with your other leg. This is 1 set. Repeat until you've done 2 sets of 8 repetitions with each leg.

Notes from your personal trainer:

You'll feel the effort in your outer hip and the thigh of your top leg. Try to keep your body in a straight line; don't lean forward or back. And keep your toes pointing forward, not up! At first, you may not be able to lift your leg more than a foot off the ground. But your range of motion will increase over time. Eventually, you may be able to lift your leg so that it forms a 45-degree angle with the floor—that's as high as it should go.

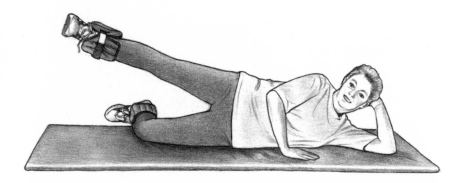

EXERCISE 8A: ANKLE EXERCISE 1—
Standing calf and toe raise ◆

As women get older, their ankles often become weaker and less flexible—which adds to the risk of falling. This exercise increases lower-leg strength and ankle flexibility, so it helps improve balance. Once you've mastered the first version, you can switch to the second for added challenge.

Starting position: Stand facing a counter or wall, about 6 to 12 inches away, with your feet hip-width apart. Place your fingertips lightly on the counter or wall for balance. Stand tall, with your knees slightly bent and your chest and head lifted.

1-2-3-Up: Slowly raise yourself up as high as possible on the balls of your feet.

Hold for three seconds and take a breath.

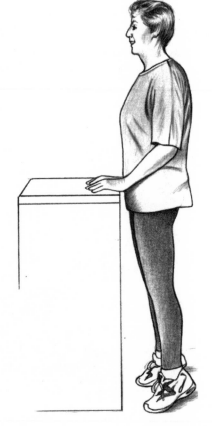

1-2-3-Down: Slowly lower yourself back to the starting position.

Reps and sets: Perform the sequence 8 times—that's 1 set. Rest a minute. During this rest, slowly raise the balls of your feet up as high as possible, so that you are standing on your heels. Don't lean backward or lock your knees. Then do a second set of 8 reps.

Notes from your personal trainer:

You'll feel the effort in your calves and shins. Try to keep your torso as erect as possible—resist the tendency to lean forward while standing on your heels. Keep your knees slightly bent so they're not locked.

As soon as you can easily get your heels at least 3 inches off the ground when doing the toe stand, and your toes 2 inches off the ground when you stand on your heels, try the second version, which is more challenging—and ultimately more beneficial.

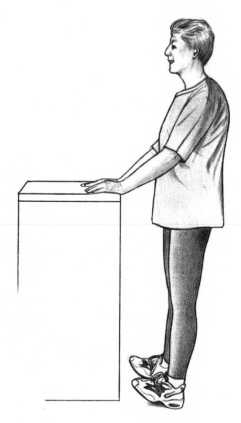

EXERCISE 8B: ANKLE EXERCISE 2—
Push and pull toes ◆

You'll further strengthen your calves and ankles with this more advanced version of the exercise. Strong lower legs mean you can climb
steps with less effort, walk more easily, and keep your balance better.

Starting position: Sit in a chair with your feet flat on the floor. The
seat of the chair should be deep enough to support your entire thigh. Strap
the ankle weights snugly around your feet so they rest on top of your
shoelaces. Position yourself so your back is against the back of the chair.
Place your hands on your thighs and extend your legs slightly so your heels
are 3 to 4 inches off the floor.

1-2-3-Push: While keeping your legs raised off the floor, push your toes
away from you as far as you can. Your legs should not
move.

Pause for a breath with your toes pointed away from
your body.

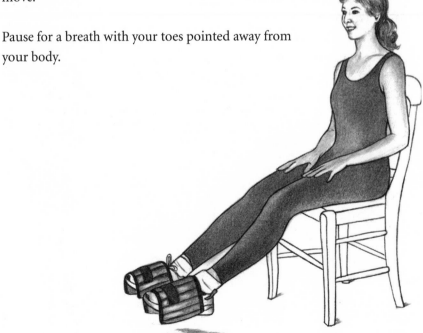

1-2-3-Pull: Pull your toes toward you as much as you can. Your legs should not move.

Pause for a breath, then repeat the move.

Reps and sets: Alternate pushing and pulling your toes for a total of 8 times in each direction. Rest for a minute or two with your feet on the floor. Lift your feet again and do a second set of 8 reps.

Notes from your personal trainer:

You'll feel the move in your shins, calves, and ankles—the entire lower leg. Because your quadriceps are working to keep your legs raised off the floor, you will feel the move in your thighs. However, you should not feel any effort in your knees. If you do, check that they're slightly bent and not locked, and that your feet are just a few inches off the floor.

Don't try to advance too quickly. If your thighs are too uncomfortable, lower your legs so they're only 2 inches off the floor while you do the move. Or rest after 4 reps if you need a break. If your feet wobble or rotate out to the side as you flex them, decrease the weight by a pound or two.

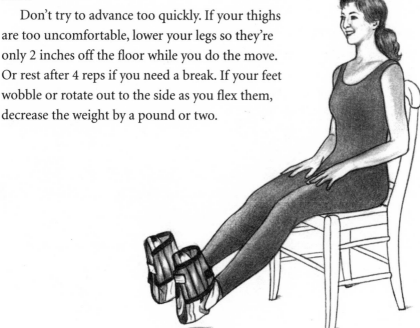

WEEK 12 AND THEREAFTER

Add the last two exercises, bringing the total to ten. To further increase the value of your workout, substitute the front lunge for the wide leg squat as your first exercise.

EXERCISE 9: CHEST PRESS ◆

Strong chest muscles contribute to good posture and a strong back. This exercise strengthens your chest muscles (under your breasts), the front of your shoulders, and the back of your arms. These muscles help support your breasts and are important for pushing and lifting motions.

Starting position: Place your dumbbells on the floor far enough apart so you can lie between them. Lie down on the floor with your knees bent, feet flat on the floor approximately hip-width apart. Carefully pick up the dumbbells. Move your upper arms out to the sides of your body so they are resting on the floor. Raise your forearms straight up and parallel to each other like goalposts. Your palms should face your feet, with your wrists and elbows in a straight line. Position the dumbbells in line with your midchest.

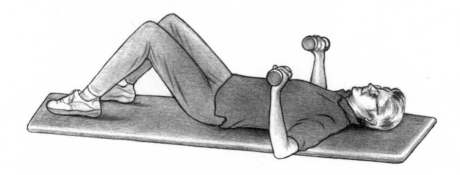

1-2-3-Up: Press the dumbbells straight up so that your arms are fully extended with your wrists, elbows, and shoulders in a straight line. Your elbows should not be locked.

Pause for a breath.

1-2-3-Down: Slowly lower the dumbbells back to the starting position.

Pause for a breath, then repeat the move. The small of your back should remain on the floor while you complete the set.

Reps and sets: Repeat until you have done 8 reps—this is 1 set. Rest for a minute or two and do a second set.

Notes from your personal trainer:

You'll feel the effort in your chest and shoulders, as well as in your forearm and the back of your upper arm. Make sure your neck and shoulders remain relaxed. A common error is to let the dumbbells drift in toward your chest and up toward your neck—check that they're at chest level and out to the side. Also be sure to keep your wrists straight.

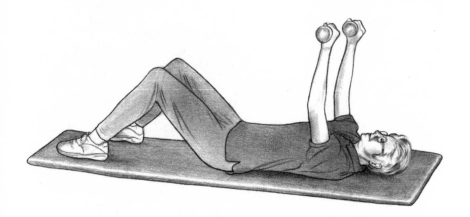

EXERCISE 10: BICEPS CURL WITH ROTATION ◆

The group of muscles in the front of your upper arm is called the biceps muscles. They bend the elbow joint and rotate your forearm. Strengthening these muscles increases the density of the wrist bone, a common site for osteoporotic fractures. An added benefit: This exercise will help you carry heavy loads with ease.

Starting position: Sit toward the front of the chair with your feet flat on the floor about hip-width apart. Hold a dumbbell in each hand so that your elbows and upper arms are snug against the sides of your body. Your forearms should be extended straight down at your sides with your palms facing your thighs.

1-2-3-Up: Raise the dumbbell in one hand toward your shoulder by bringing your forearm up. Rotate your forearm in a smooth motion as you lift the dumbbell, so that your thumb turns toward the outside of your body. Your palm should be directly in front of and facing your shoulder in the lifted position. Your elbow remains in the same position throughout the move—it does not come forward.

Pause for a breath.

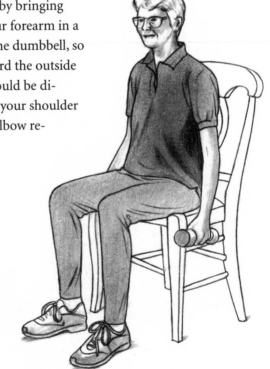

1-2-3-Down: Slowly lower the dumbbell and rotate your forearm to return to the starting position.

Pause for a breath, then repeat the move with your other arm.

Reps and sets: Repeat the move, alternating arms, until you have done 8 repetitions with each arm. That's 1 set. Rest and do a second set.

Notes from your personal trainer:

You'll feel the effort in the front of your upper arm and forearm. Keep your elbows in the proper position by imagining that you're holding a newspaper against your body with each arm. Check your wrist at the top of each lift to make sure it's not bent—it should remain in line with the rest of the forearm.

For efficiency, you can do the move with both arms simultaneously. However, some people arch their back when they attempt to perform two-handed biceps curls. So working one arm at a time is safer even if it's a little slower. Another advantage is that you can lift more weight with each arm, thereby getting greater benefit from the exercise.

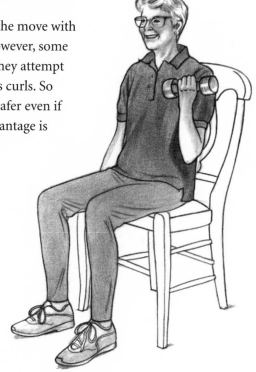

NEW EXERCISE 1: FRONT LUNGE ◆

After twelve weeks you can substitute this exercise for the wide leg squat. The lunge is a dynamic exercise that targets the muscles of the thighs, back, and buttocks, strengthening the bones in the hip and spine. The wide leg squat addresses the same muscles, but the lunge includes balance and coordination as well.

Starting position: Stand next to a table or counter with your feet hip-width apart, knees slightly bent. Lightly hold on to the counter with one hand.

1-2-3-Forward: Take a large step forward with your right leg. Land on the heel of your right foot, then roll your foot forward until it is flat on the floor. Keeping your body erect, bend both knees so that your hips drop straight down. Your front thigh should be almost parallel to the floor, and the knee of your back leg should approach the floor. The knee of your for-

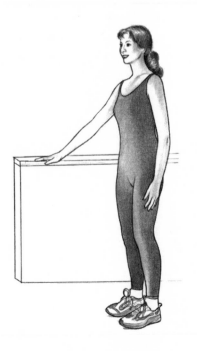
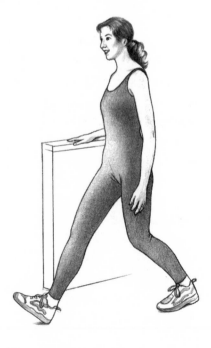

ward leg should be over your ankle, not past your toes. The heel of your back leg will come off the floor. Your weight will be equally distributed between your front foot and the ball of your back foot.

Pause for a breath.

Return: Push back forcefully with the front leg to return to the starting position.

Pause for a breath, then repeat the move.

Reps and sets: Alternate legs as you step forward until you have done 8 reps with each leg—this is 1 set. Rest for a minute or two and do a second set.

Notes from your personal trainer:

You'll feel the effort in your thighs, buttocks, and back. Keep your body erect. In the forward move, concentrate on dropping your hips straight down. Push backward, not upward, when returning to the starting position. If you feel the effort in the knee of the leading leg, your knee probably is moving in front of your toes rather than remaining directly above your ankle.

    To increase the challenge once you've mastered this exercise, work toward doing the move without holding on with your hands. When that becomes too easy, hold a dumbbell in each hand to increase the effort.

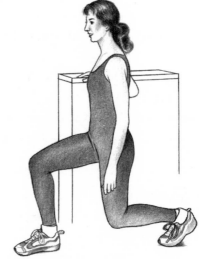

Creating an individualized strength-training program

Maintaining the right challenge is the secret of both safety and success. If you overdo it, you'll find the program unnecessarily difficult. On the other hand, if you expect too little of yourself, you won't see the kind of progress that makes strength training so exciting.

Where to start

I suggest you begin very conservatively, with weights that are easy to lift. This allows you to focus on your form. Later, as your muscles strengthen, you'll add weight or switch to the harder version of the exercise. That way the program will always be right for your body. Use these guidelines to select a starting weight:

- If you have established osteoporosis or other health concerns, discuss the program with your doctor before you begin. One option to discuss with your doctor is beginning the exercises without weights.
- If you've never strength-trained before (or haven't done so recently) and are in good health, begin with 3-pound weights. If that's uncomfortable, use 1-pound weights, or begin with no weights.
- If you're already following another strength-training program but want to switch to the exercises in this book, start with weights that are the same or lower than what you're using now. For a familiar exercise, use your customary weight; if the exercise is new, use your lightest weight and increase after a session or two.

How to evaluate your effort

This scale—inspired by the Borg Exercise Intensity Scale that many researchers use—will help you determine if you're working out at the right intensity.

Aim to work out at level 4. You should find the weight moderately difficult to lift the first time, but well within your capability. By the third or fourth lift, it should seem heavier. Ideally, you should be able to perform the eighth lift in good form, but feel that if you didn't stop and rest your muscles, you couldn't continue.

Working out at level 3 (except for the first week or two) is not sufficiently

EXERCISE-INTENSITY SCALE FOR STRENGTH TRAINING	
EXERCISE INTENSITY	DESCRIPTION OF EFFORT
1	*Very easy:* Too easy to be noticed, like lifting a pencil.
2	*Easy:* Can be felt but isn't fatiguing, like carrying a book.
3	*Moderate:* Fatiguing only if prolonged—like carrying a full handbag that seems heavier as the day goes on.
4	*Hard:* More than moderate at first, and becoming difficult by the time you complete four or five repetitions. You can make the effort eight times in good form, but need to rest afterwards.
5	*Extremely hard:* Requires all your strength, like lifting a piece of heavy furniture that you can lift only once, if at all.

challenging; it will increase your endurance, but not your strength. On the other hand, training at level 5 is risky—if the effort is too great, you won't be able to maintain proper form and you might injure yourself.

With the exercises that use body weight, you won't be able to adjust your effort quite so precisely. Advance to the more difficult version as soon as you can do so without exceeding level 4 intensity. If you aren't sure, wait. It's better to progress a little more slowly than to work your muscles too hard.

Finding the right challenge

Stay at the starting level for the first two weeks to learn the exercises, even if it's too easy. If your first session seems too hard, or if your muscles are very uncomfortable afterwards, do the exercises without weights.

During the third week, for the exercises that use dumbbells, move up to the next dumbbell, as needed to increase effort to level 4. However, if your muscles become sore, continue with the same weight or, if the discomfort is bothersome, decrease the weight. You may find that you need to add weights on some exercises but not others. That's normal, because the strength of different muscles varies. Aim to reach level 4 on all the exercises by the end of the fourth or fifth week.

During the second month, try to increase the weight for each exercise every other week. That may not always be possible. Also, you'll soon see that progress is easier with some exercises than with others. Don't be discouraged—all of your muscle groups will become stronger if you persist.

Working toward goals

The following table shows strength goals by age and exercise. Most women reach these goals after a year on this program, or at least come close. However, the goals are by no means upper limits. Studies that follow people for as long as two years find that they keep improving, though of course the changes become very slow. Remember, if you have osteoporosis, talk with your doctor to determine appropriate goals for you.

When you're training at these levels, you will have obtained most of the bone and other health benefits you can expect from a strengthening program—provided you keep it up. How much farther you go is up to you. But don't go above 20 pounds with the ankle weights or above 25 pounds with dumbbells, since using heavier free weights could create joint problems. My personal preference is to maintain healthy levels and vary the routine periodically, rather than struggling to lift ever heavier weights.

◆ ◆ ◆

I have such small wrists, and there's arthritis in my family. Also, I'd had a frozen shoulder before. So I went at strength training very carefully. It took me two years to get to 9 pounds. Strength training helped me a lot— it strengthened my left side where I had surgery for breast cancer fifteen years ago.

—NAN, AGE 63, WHO HAS OSTEOPOROSIS

◆ ◆ ◆

STRENGTH-TRAINING GOALS			
EXERCISE	20 TO 49 YEARS OLD	50 TO 69 YEARS OLD	70 YEARS AND OLDER
Wide leg squat	Work toward not touching the chair and add 5- to 10-pound dumbbells	Work toward not touching the chair and add 5- to 8-pound dumbbells	Work toward not touching the chair
Step up	Two steps, with 5- to 8-pound dumbbells	Two steps, with 3- to 5-pound dumbbells	Two steps
Seated overhead press	8 to 12 pounds	5 to 10 pounds	5 to 8 pounds
Forward fly	8 to 12 pounds	5 to 8 pounds	3 to 5 pounds
Back extension	Chest and thigh off the floor	Chest and thigh off the floor	Chest and thigh off the floor
Abdominal exercise	Reverse curl	Reverse curl	Reverse curl
Side leg raise	8 to 12 pounds	5 to 10 pounds	3 to 8 pounds
Ankle exercise	Push and pull toes with 15- to 20-pound ankle weights	Push and pull toes with 10- to 15-pound ankle weights	Push and pull toes with 5- to 10-pound ankle weights
Chest press	12 to 20 pounds	10 to 15 pounds	5 to 8 pounds
Biceps curl with rotation	10 to 15 pounds	8 to 12 pounds	5 to 10 pounds
Front lunge	Controlled and with good balance, using 5- to 10-pound dumbbells	Controlled and with good balance, using 3- to 5-pound dumbbells	Controlled and with good balance
Wrist curl	5 to 8 pounds	3 to 5 pounds	1 to 3 pounds

Strength training at a health club

Some women prefer to exercise at a fitness center or gym. Indeed, a health club has advantages, especially for those with medical problems who need closer supervision: Personal trainers are available; they can help you customize your program to match your needs and limitations. If you have osteopenia or osteoporosis, there's another plus to consider: working out on a machine—which holds you in the correct position—allows you to safely lift more weight, thereby giving more stimulation to your bones.

Here are some suggestions if you'd like to do your strength training on machines at a gym:

- Follow the basic recommendations about exercise intensity, the number of reps and sets, and how to progress.
- Ask a trainer to show you how to adjust the equipment so that it fits you—that's essential for safety and effectiveness.
- Select exercises that target the major muscle groups of the body plus areas particularly vulnerable to osteoporosis—the spine, the hips, and the wrists. A good program will probably include:

  Leg press
  Hip abduction
  Hip adduction
  Knee extension
  Knee curl (sometimes called hamstring curl)
  Lat pull-down
  Chest press
  Overhead press
  Upper back (sometime called seated row)

- If you have osteoporosis or back problems, be particularly careful about using abdominal and back-extension machines. Ask the trainer for instructions.
- Include the following exercises from this book because they improve coordination and trunk strength:

  Step up
  Abdominal exercise

Back extension

Ankle exercise

Lunge

- Don't hesitate to ask for help—that's one of the benefits of working out at a health club.

To readers of *Strong Women Stay Young* and *Strong Women Stay Slim*

If you've read one or both of my other books, you may be puzzled to see that the exercises in this book are different. Perhaps you're wondering which program to follow. Here are explanations and recommendations:

- *Strong Women Stay Young* aims to strengthen muscles in the arms, legs, and trunk of the body. The exercises also benefit bones and improve balance.
- *Strong Women Stay Slim* offers information and instructions for healthy weight loss, including a streamlined strength-training program, aerobic exercise, and a food plan based on the Food Guide Pyramid.
- *Strong Women, Strong Bones* focuses on osteoporosis, with a comprehensive exercise program that includes strengthening exercises designed to promote bone health. This is the best program to use if you're particularly concerned about your bones.

If you're using the exercises in one of my books and prefer to continue with them, you can do so. But for optimal health and fitness, I urge you to include aerobic and balance exercises—as well as vertical jumping if appropriate—in your workouts. Also, I suggest you add or swap at least some of the strengthening exercises from this book. Variety benefits your body and keeps your strength-training sessions interesting.

Follow these guidelines when you create new strengthening workouts:

- Start with a warm-up. A chair stand is excellent for this purpose.
- Select a variety of exercises that work the major muscles in the arms, legs, and trunk. To avoid overworking a muscle, use just one version of an exercise (for instance, do either a biceps curl from one of the other books or the biceps curl with rotation from this book, but not both). Remember that the exercises in this book are best if you have osteoporosis or back problems.
- Finish with a cool-down and stretch.

BALANCE EXERCISES

Balance exercises actually tax your brain more than your muscles. Their important contribution to bone health is to help prevent falls. With just a little physical effort, you can make significant progress very quickly. In fact, the worse your balance is now, the faster you'll improve. Research shows that balance training can reduce falls in older men and women by about 50 percent. Changes won't be as dramatic if your balance is already good, but I hope you'll do the exercises anyway—better balance is helpful at any age.

General instructions

We usually keep our feet hip-width apart when we walk—a wide base makes balance easier. Balance exercises do just the opposite: they challenge your balancing ability by creating a narrow base of support. Though the exercises are safe if you do them carefully, it's important to observe simple cautions:

- If you scored "poor" or "very poor" on the balance test in Chapter 6 (see page 87), it is essential that you have a spotter nearby when you perform these exercises. Discuss your balance problems with your doctor—sometimes there's a treatable cause.

- If your balance is impaired by an illness that affects your ears, such as a bad cold, or by a medication, skip these exercises until you're better.
- Wear sturdy shoes when you do the exercises.
- Perform the moves near a counter, with one hand poised to catch yourself if necessary.
- If you find yourself teetering, stop. Regain your balance before you start again.

THE EXERCISES

Aim to do the balance exercises at least three times per week, after your strength-training workout. They're a great way to cool down. But if you enjoy them, you can do them as frequently as you'd like. They don't require a warm-up or cool-down.

MOUNTAIN POSE AND SWAY ◆

This exercise has been adapted from a classic yoga pose, and is designed to improve your body awareness, which helps prevent falls. Improved body awareness—your brain's ability to know exactly where all parts of your body are in space—is helpful with both balance and coordination. The mountain pose is an excellent cool-down exercise and a wonderful stress reliever, since it has a very calming effect on the body.

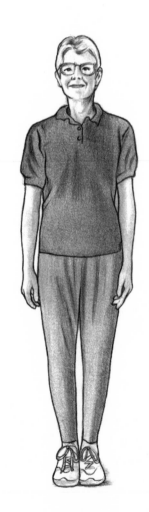

Position: Stand with your feet close together, touching if possible, knees slightly bent. Distribute your body weight evenly between the balls and heels of your feet. Keep your arms straight down at your sides, with your hands relaxed. Your shoulders should be down and gently drawn back; your head should be high. Tuck the bones of your pelvis under—moving them slightly forward and up.

Working up from the soles of your feet, visualize how each part of your body rises from the part below it. Sense how your shinbones rise from your feet to your knees. Notice how the slight bend of your knees allows your thigh and hip bones to extend up in neutral alignment. Feel your rib cage expanding and lifting. Sense how the vertebras of your spine stack upon each other. Imagine that the spaces between the vertebras are expanding, lengthening your spine. Your head should feel almost weightless and you should feel slightly taller than before the pose.

Hold this position for a minimum of thirty seconds up to two minutes, breathing evenly.

To increase the challenge: After holding the position for at least thirty seconds, add postural sway. Visualize the soles of both feet anchored to the ground. Very slowly move your entire body slightly forward, then slightly to the left, to the back and then to the right and to the front again. The full circle (forward, left, back, right, forward) should take about one minute to complete. During the sway, your entire body should remain re-laxed and straight. Don't bend at the hip or back—only your ankles should bend.

Release the pose: Step one foot out to the side so that your feet are hip-width apart.

Notes from your personal trainer:

Your entire body should feel relaxed. If you feel unsteady initially, widen your stance a little. Concentrate on the soles of your feet. During the sway, you will feel your weight move to the balls of your feet, then to the outside of your left foot, then to your heels, to the outside of your right foot, and then back again onto the balls of your feet. This is a difficult move. At first, your body will move only a few inches from the center as you do the sway. But over time, you will improve.

ONE-LEGGED STORK ◆

This exercise also is adapted from a classic yoga pose. It's designed to improve your posture, your balance, and the flexibility of your hip.

Position: Stand to the side of a counter or wall with your feet hip-width apart. Your knees should be slightly bent. Hold the counter or touch the wall lightly with one hand for support; hold your other arm straight out to the side. Bring one knee up slightly, about 6 inches, keeping your back straight. Point the toes of that foot down and turn your knee out to the side by rotating your hip. Place the bottom of your foot against your opposite shin. Keep your head up and your eyes focused on a location straight ahead.

Hold this position for a minimum of thirty seconds, up to two minutes.

Release the pose: Lower your knee and return to the starting position.

Reps: Perform the move once with each leg.

Notes from your personal trainer:

You'll feel the effort in the leg that you're standing on and in the hip of the lifted leg. This is a challenging move. Be patient with yourself and progress slowly. Try to lift your knee higher and balance with your hand poised near the counter or wall instead of holding on.

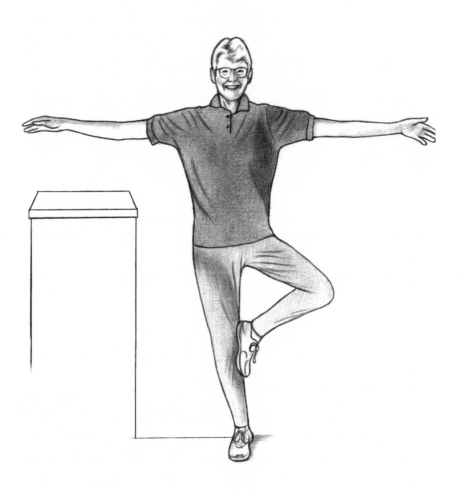

TANDEM WALK ◆

Police use the tandem walk to test for drunk driving—it's nearly impossible to perform a tandem walk if your balance and coordination are compromised by alcohol. Though the test is very helpful for those with poor balance, it's not sufficiently challenging for those with good balance. Add it to your exercise program only if you scored 3 or less on the balance test in Chapter 6.

Starting position: Find a hallway with a clear wall where you can walk at least ten to twenty steps while holding on to the wall. Place one hand on the wall at shoulder height for support. Focus your eyes on a location straight ahead. Keep your head up and don't look at your feet.

The move: Place one foot in front of the other so that the heel of your front foot touches the toes of your back foot, forming a straight line. Don't lock your knees. Walk toe to heel in tandem style for approximately ten to twenty steps. Move your hand along the wall to help you remain balanced. Turn around carefully and walk back again, toe to heel, for ten to twenty steps.

Reps: Repeat the walk two times.

Notes from your personal trainer:

Try not to look at your feet. Instead, feel your heel and toes touch as you walk, and concentrate on letting your feet form a straight line. To increase the challenge: Don't touch the wall as you walk, but keep your hand poised to recover your balance if necessary.

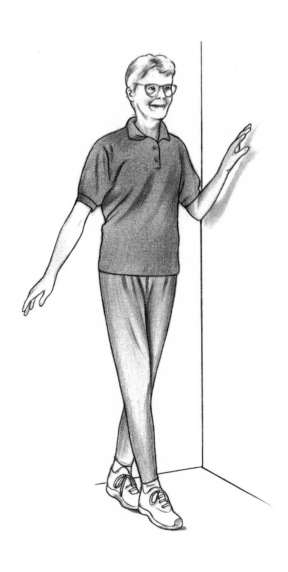

STRETCHING

Stretching is a vital component of any exercise program. A brief stretch after your workout is a wonderful way to relax—and it helps prevent injury and maintain flexibility. Furthermore, stretching helps reduce back pain from osteoporosis, as well as other aches and pains.

General instructions

Stretching is necessary after you strength-train or do aerobic exercise. But you can stretch as often as you please. A stretch is one of my favorite pick-me-ups when I'm working at my computer. I take a two-minute stretch break every hour to remove the tension from my neck, back, and shoulders—it's a real revitalizer that makes me feel good all over. The basics couldn't be easier:

- **Get into position:** Extend your muscles as far as you comfortably can.
- **Hold the stretch:** Breathe normally and hold the stretch for twenty to thirty seconds. Gently try to extend the position, but never bounce or go to the point of discomfort. Try to relax your muscles as much as possible—the more you relax, the more your muscles will be able to stretch.
- **Release:** Slowly release the stretch and return to a normal position.

THE STRETCHES

Do these stretches at the end of every exercise session. If you combine your weight-bearing and strength training in a single workout, do one set of stretches after strength training. I also encourage you to stretch whenever you need to relax and relieve tension.

◆   ◆   ◆

I have osteoporosis. I work on posture all the time, because the only thing that relieves pain from the crushed vertebra is perfect posture. Also, I've lost a fraction of an inch of height.

In addition to going to the fitness club three times a week, I exercise every day for fifteen to twenty minutes early in the morning. I jog on tiptoe for ten minutes, and then I do a lot of stretching. I used to have trouble getting going in the morning, but this wakes me up. And I'm not bent over.

—ANNE

◆   ◆   ◆

HAMSTRING STRETCH ◆

You'll need a towel for this stretch, which improves the flexibility of the hamstring muscles in the backs of your thighs as well as your lower back. It promotes flexibility of the back, reducing the risk of injury and also relieving and preventing lower back pain. This exercise is safe—and very beneficial—for women with osteoporosis.

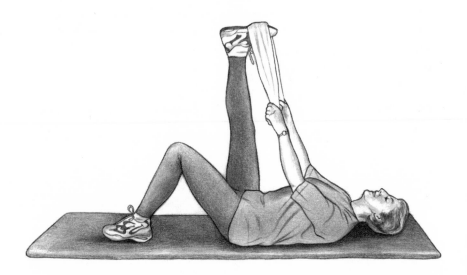

Starting position: Lie on your back on the floor, holding the ends of a towel in your hands. Your knees should be bent with your feet flat on the floor; the small of your back should be pressed against the floor. Bend one knee toward you and loop the towel around the bottom of your shoe. Extend this leg straight up so the sole of your shoe is flat and facing the ceiling. Your knee should not be locked. The towel will help you maintain the correct position.

The stretch: Slowly pull on both ends of the towel to draw your leg toward your body until you feel a gentle stretch. The leg may move just an inch or several inches, depending on your flexibility. Keep your buttocks on the mat. Also, be sure to keep the foot of the stretched leg flat—if you point your toe toward the ceiling, the stretch won't be as effective. Hold the stretch for twenty to thirty seconds, breathing normally and relaxing the rest of your body. Then release.

Reps: Perform 1 stretch with each leg. Repeat if desired. You'll feel the stretch along the back of your thigh and calf.

SHOULDER STRETCH ◆

This stretch will help improve your posture and the flexibility of your back—plus it's a great tension reliever.

Starting position: Stand with your feet hip-width apart, knees slightly bent and shoulder blades drawn slightly together in the back. Lace your fingers together and then rotate your wrists so that your palms face away from you. Press your palms out and away from your body, until your arms are straight but unlocked. Keeping your shoulders down and back, lift your arms up to chest height.

The stretch: Press your palms away from you until you feel gentle tension across your back and shoulders. Don't bend your spine forward when you do this exercise. Also, be sure not to lock your elbows. Check for tension in your neck—your entire body, except for the parts you're stretching, should be relaxed. Hold the stretch for twenty to thirty seconds, breathing normally.

Reps: Perform 1 stretch. Repeat if desired. You'll feel the stretch across your back, shoulders, and arms.

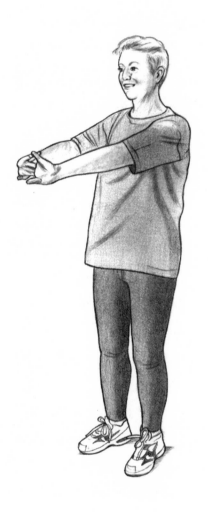

UPPER BACK PULLBACK ◆

This is a particularly helpful exercise for women with osteoporosis, back pain, or curvature of the spine. It stretches out the muscles of your chest and the middle of your upper back, improving posture and relieving pain. You can perform this stretch any time you're sitting down. I do it hourly when I'm sitting at my desk.

Starting position: Sit toward the front of your chair with your feet flat on the floor and hip-width apart. Bend your elbows so that your forearms are parallel to your thighs and your upper arms are against the sides of your body.

The stretch: Press your shoulders down and draw your shoulder blades together in back. Your upper arms will move back slightly. Sit with good posture and hold the stretch for twenty to thirty seconds, breathing normally and relaxing the rest of your body. Pause for a moment and then repeat a second time if desired.

Reps: Perform 1 stretch. Repeat if desired. You'll feel the stretch across your chest and back.

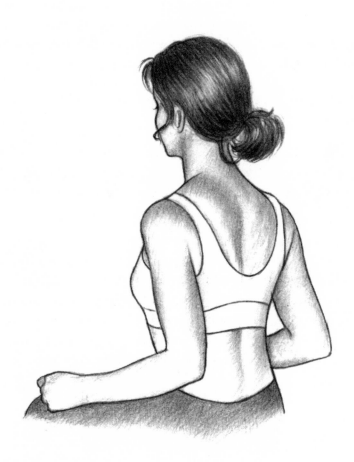

WHAT TO EXPECT DURING THE FIRST TWELVE WEEKS

It's always exciting—and sometimes a little overwhelming—to make important lifestyle changes. During the first twelve weeks of this program, you'll become significantly fitter and stronger. I urge you to fill in the exercise log on page 264. They will help you stay on track. Later you'll enjoy rereading your early entries and marveling at the improvements.

Planning your workouts

Some women prefer to spread their exercise over the entire week; others like to schedule fewer but longer workouts. Either way is fine. Below are two possibilities—but I want to emphasize that there are many others. The best system is the one you can stick to.

A three-day option

If you want to do aerobic exercise and strength training on the same day, follow this sequence—it assures that your muscles are properly warmed up at the beginning and cooled down at the end. Allow at least one day between strength-training workouts to give your muscles time to rest. But feel free to do extra aerobic activity, vertical jumping, balance exercises, and stretches on your "off" days.

- Weight-bearing aerobic activity (start slowly to warm up)
- Vertical jumping (if appropriate)
- Strength training
- Balance exercises
- Stretches

A six-day option

Three days a week you'll follow this sequence to complete your aerobic workouts:

- Weight-bearing aerobic activity (start slowly to warm up)
- Vertical jumping (if appropriate)
- Balance exercises
- Stretches

On alternate days your workouts will include strength training instead of weight-bearing aerobic exercise:

- Vertical jumping (if appropriate)
- Strength training
- Balance exercises
- Stretches

If time is short, you can reduce vertical jumping and balance exercises to three times a week.

Weeks 1 to 3

Most women I work with see a difference almost immediately, especially if they've been sedentary. First, they feel good about themselves for starting to exercise. They experience a postexercise lift, and often tell me they have more energy throughout the day and sleep better at night.

WEEKS 1–3: THREE-DAY OPTION							
EXERCISE	SUN	MON	TUE	WED	THU	FRI	SAT
Aerobic activity (minutes)		15		15		15	
Vertical jumping (if appropriate)		✓		✓		✓	
Strength training							
Wide leg squat		✓		✓		✓	
Step up		✓		✓		✓	
Seated overhead press		✓		✓		✓	
Forward fly		✓		✓		✓	
Balance exercises		✓		✓		✓	
Stretches		✓		✓		✓	

WEEKS 1–3: SIX-DAY OPTION							
EXERCISE	SUN	MON	TUE	WED	THU	FRI	SAT
Aerobic activity (minutes)	15		15		15		
Vertical jumping (if appropriate)	✓	✓	✓	✓	✓	✓	
Strength training							
Wide leg squat		✓		✓		✓	
Step up		✓		✓		✓	
Seated overhead press		✓		✓		✓	
Forward fly		✓		✓		✓	
Balance exercises	✓	✓	✓	✓	✓	✓	
Stretches	✓	✓	✓	✓	✓	✓	

Weeks 4 to 7

By now your workouts should be familiar and comfortable. Indeed, I hope they're so enjoyable that you actually miss them if you have to skip a session. To maintain level 3 effort in your aerobic activity, you've probably stepped up the pace—you're walking a little faster, playing tennis more vigorously. In your strength training, you should be lifting weights at level 4 intensity. In the second month, you may be lifting *twice* as much weight as you did at the beginning.

WEEKS 4-7: THREE-DAY OPTION							
EXERCISE	SUN	MON	TUE	WED	THU	FRI	SAT
Aerobic activity (minutes)		20		20		20	
Vertical jumping (if appropriate)		✓		✓		✓	
Strength training							
Wide leg squat		✓		✓		✓	
Step up		✓		✓		✓	
Seated overhead press		✓		✓		✓	
Forward fly		✓		✓		✓	
Back extension		✓		✓		✓	
Abdominal exercise		✓		✓		✓	
Balance exercises		✓		✓		✓	
Stretches		✓		✓		✓	

WEEKS 4-7: SIX-DAY OPTION							
EXERCISE	SUN	MON	TUE	WED	THU	FRI	SAT
Aerobic activity (minutes)	20		20		20		
Vertical jumping (if appropriate)	✓	✓	✓	✓	✓	✓	
Strength training							
Wide leg squat		✓		✓		✓	
Step up		✓		✓		✓	
Seated overhead press		✓		✓		✓	
Forward fly		✓		✓		✓	
Back extension		✓		✓		✓	
Abdominal exercise							
Balance exercises	✓	✓	✓	✓	✓	✓	
Stretches	✓	✓	✓	✓	✓	✓	

Weeks 8 to 11

As you start the third month, you're probably enjoying many payoffs: increased energy and stamina, a more toned appearance, better balance, greater flexibility. All this is evidence that your body is getting fitter.

WEEKS 8–11: THREE-DAY OPTION							
EXERCISE	SUN	MON	TUE	WED	THU	FRI	SAT
Aerobic activity (minutes)		25		25		25	
Vertical jumping (if appropriate)		✓		✓		✓	
Strength training							
Wide leg squat		✓		✓		✓	
Step up		✓		✓		✓	
Seated overhead press		✓		✓		✓	
Forward fly		✓		✓		✓	
Back extension		✓		✓		✓	
Abdominal exercise		✓		✓		✓	
Side leg raise		✓		✓		✓	
Ankle exercise		✓		✓		✓	
Balance exercises		✓		✓		✓	
Stretches		✓		✓		✓	

WEEKS 8–11: SIX-DAY OPTION							
EXERCISE	SUN	MON	TUE	WED	THU	FRI	SAT
Aerobic activity (minutes)	25		25		25		
Vertical jumping (if appropriate)	✓	✓	✓	✓	✓	✓	
Strength training							
Wide leg squat		✓		✓		✓	
Step up		✓		✓		✓	
Seated overhead press		✓		✓		✓	
Forward fly		✓		✓		✓	
Back extension		✓		✓		✓	
Abdominal exercise		✓		✓		✓	
Side leg raise		✓		✓		✓	
Ankle exercise		✓		✓		✓	
Balance exercises	✓	✓	✓	✓	✓	✓	
Stretches	✓	✓	✓	✓	✓	✓	

Week 12 and thereafter

Congratulations! You're exercising thirty minutes three to six days a week—which puts you in the most active quarter of American women. Depending on where you started, your cardiovascular fitness has probably increased by 10 to 20 percent, and the amount of weight you can lift has probably tripled! What's more, you've developed an exercise habit that will keep you fit. Your bones are starting to change, but they need time—at least a year—for the difference to be large enough to see.

WEEKS 12 AND THEREAFTER: THREE-DAY OPTION							
EXERCISE	SUN	MON	TUE	WED	THU	FRI	SAT
Aerobic activity (minutes)		30		30		30	
Vertical jumping (if appropriate)		✓		✓		✓	
Strength training							
Front lunge or squat		✓		✓		✓	
Step up		✓		✓		✓	
Seated overhead press		✓		✓		✓	
Forward fly		✓		✓		✓	
Back extension		✓		✓		✓	
Abdominal exercise		✓		✓		✓	
Side leg raise		✓		✓		✓	
Ankle exercise		✓		✓		✓	
Chest press		✓		✓		✓	
Biceps curl with rotation		✓		✓		✓	
Balance exercises		✓		✓		✓	
Stretches		✓		✓		✓	

EXERCISE	SUN	MON	TUE	WED	Thu	FRI	SAT
WEEKS 12 AND THEREAFTER: SIX-DAY OPTION							
Aerobic activity (minutes)	30		30		30		
Vertical jumping (if appropriate)	✓	✓	✓	✓	✓	✓	
Strength training							
Front lunge or squat		✓		✓		✓	
Step up		✓		✓		✓	
Seated overhead press		✓		✓		✓	
Forward fly		✓		✓		✓	
Back extension		✓		✓		✓	
Abdominal exercise		✓		✓		✓	
Side leg raise		✓		✓		✓	
Ankle exercise		✓		✓		✓	
Chest press		✓		✓		✓	
Biceps curl with rotation							
Balance exercises	✓	✓	✓	✓	✓	✓	
Stretches	✓	✓	✓	✓	✓	✓	

What's next?

Now that your exercise habit is firmly established, it's a good idea to vary activities. New exercises stimulate other muscles and bones, and they keep your workouts interesting.

Some women are willing to invest the time in longer aerobic workouts. That's fine—just be sure to increase gradually, adding no more than five minutes to your workout in a week. For example, take at least three weeks to increase your workouts from thirty to forty-five minutes.

After about six to nine months of strength training, you'll probably reach the goals on page 195. Any further advances will come much more slowly. I believe that it's more beneficial for bone to add new exercises than to struggle to improve further.

I hope you'll explore other forms of exercise, such as yoga and Tai Chi, as well as active pastimes like ballroom dancing and fencing. There are so many possibilities for enjoying physical activity!

> *"If doctors could prescribe exercise in pill form, it would be the single most widely prescribed drug in the world."*
> —ROBERT BUTLER, M.D., FOUNDING DIRECTOR OF THE NATIONAL INSTITUTE ON AGING

Despite all the miraculous inventions of modern medicine, there's still no single intervention that can improve your overall health more than physical activity. An active lifestyle that includes the exercises in this chapter also will benefit your bones and protect you from fractures.

As you finish this long chapter, I hope you're enthusiastic about starting— but I'm a little concerned that you may feel overwhelmed. Begin slowly; progress gradually. You'll get there! What's important for your bones is not what happens in an hour or a day, but consistency over weeks, months, and years.

Fitness information resources

Organization
Shape-Up America! (a program started by C. Everett Koop, M.D.)
6707 Democracy Boulevard, Suite 306; Bethesda, MD 20817;
301/493-5368
http://www.shapeup.org

Books
Biomarkers: The 10 Determinants of Aging You Can Control, by
William Evans, Ph.D., and Irwin Rosenberg, M.D., with Jaqueline
Thompson (Simon & Schuster, 1991)

The Wellness Guide to Lifelong Fitness, by Timothy P. White, Ph.D.,
and the editors of the University of California at Berkeley Wellness
Letter (REBUS, distributed by Random House, 1993)

Fitness and Health, by Brian Sharkey, Ph.D. (Human Kinetics, 1996)

ACSM Fitness Book, by the American College of Sports Medicine
(Human Kinetics, 1997)

Good News
About Medication

◆ ◆ ◆

In the early 1980s, when I was a graduate student reading the scientific literature about osteoporosis, estrogen was the only available treatment. Calcitonin, a bone-preserving thyroid hormone, came along in 1985. But in those days it had to be taken by injection. Women with osteoporosis had very limited choices. Then finally, in the mid-1990s, things began to change. Alendronate (brand name Fosamax) received approval from the Food and Drug Administration in 1995—the first nonhormonal treatment for bone loss. This was a major and very exciting advance. Three years later, raloxifene (brand name Evista) was approved. And this is just the beginning.

Research has expanded tremendously. Numerous promising medications are under investigation. We're also learning about the therapeutic importance of nutrition and exercise. Today there are more choices and better strategies than ever before. In just a few years the list of osteoporosis treatment and prevention measures will be even longer.

If you're at high risk for bone loss, medication can improve your odds. If you already have osteopenia or osteoporosis, medication can curb the losses and even restore bone mass. Many women stand to benefit from the exciting new pharmacological developments. But the options can be confusing. This chapter will explain current and likely future drugs—how they work and strategies for using them successfully.

A QUICK OVERVIEW

If you're diagnosed with osteopenia or osteoporosis—or if you're at very high risk—your doctor will almost certainly recommend that you do the following:

- Take a calcium supplement that includes vitamin D
- Begin (or continue) an exercise program
- Adopt fall-prevention measures (if you're at risk for falls)

The doctor may suggest one or more medications too. If you're postmenopausal, the most likely possibilities are hormone replacement therapy, raloxifene, alendronate, or calcitonin. While no medications have FDA approval for premenopausal women, doctors may prescribe alendronate or calcitonin, depending on individual circumstances.

I want to emphasize that treatment decisions are highly individual. What's right for your best friend—or even your sister—is not necessarily right for you. It's very important to make medication decisions in consultation with a knowledgeable doctor, who will consider not only your present condition but your entire medical history.

Another very important point: Drugs are *not* a substitute for good nutrition and exercise! Calcium, vitamin D, and physical activity have important therapeutic benefits all by themselves: they help maintain bone mass, and may even build bone to some extent. Also, scientists believe that osteoporosis drug treatments work best if the woman is well nourished and gets plenty of physical exercise. This assures that her body has the raw material and mechanical stimulation to make new bone.

HORMONE REPLACEMENT THERAPY

Hormone replacement therapy (HRT) is the medication most frequently prescribed for prevention and treatment of osteoporosis. I'm often asked about HRT in letters and at lectures. Women worry about taking hormones—and they also worry about *not* taking them, and possibly shortchanging their bones. It's not an easy decision, but good information helps.

How it works

As you know, estrogen plays a key role in bone health, starting from the time we enter puberty. In our mid-thirties, our ovaries begin to produce less estrogen. At age 45, as we stand on the threshold of menopause, our estrogen levels are only about 80 percent of what they were a decade earlier—and we've already begun to lose bone mass as a result. When we enter menopause, our estrogen levels plunge. At age 60, the estrogen level of the average woman is only about 12 percent of what it was when she was 35. Moreover, the remainder includes a smaller proportion of estradiol, the most potent form of estrogen. Every system in our body is affected by this change, and there's a major impact on bone.

Our bones, like most of our tissues, have special receptors for estrogen. We've known for some time that estrogen suppresses the bone-dissolving activity of the osteoclasts. Now we believe that estrogen may also stimulate the osteoblasts, the cells that build bone. In addition to these direct effects, estrogen affects bone indirectly. Here are a few of the mechanisms:

- Stimulates production of vitamin D, which helps the intestines absorb calcium
- Promotes conservation of calcium by the kidneys, so less is excreted
- Triggers release of calcitonin by the thyroid, which decreases the bone-dissolving activity of the osteoclasts
- Causes release of growth hormone by the pituitary gland, which stimulates bone formation and increases absorption of calcium in the intestines

Doctors have understood the relationship between estrogen loss and bone loss for decades. The first published paper to show that estrogen therapy helps bone was published about sixty years ago, in 1941. Since then, many careful large-scale studies have confirmed the benefits.

Treatment with estrogen alone increases the risk of uterine and endometrial cancer. Consequently, most women receive progesterone too, to counter the stimulation of the uterus by estrogen. The term "hormone replacement therapy" (HRT) refers to this combination of estrogen and progesterone. Estrogen replacement therapy (ERT) means estrogen used alone. Women whose uterus has been removed—and who therefore can't get uterine or endometrial cancer—usually are given ERT.

Women who take HRT or ERT for three to five years can expect a 50 percent reduction in their risk of spinal fractures and a 25 percent reduction in their risk of other bone fractures. Longer use of hormones (ten or more years) may lower the risk by as much as 75 percent. These benefits persist as long as a woman takes HRT or ERT. However, if she stops she can expect the same rapid bone loss that would have occurred after menopause: five to seven years later, her bone density and risk of fractures are about the same as those of a woman who never took hormones.

HRT and ERT have other important health benefits for postmenopausal women. Women who take hormones enjoy a 40 percent reduction in their risk of heart disease; research suggests they also gain some protection from Alzheimer's disease. Another benefit is easing of unpleasant symptoms of menopause, including hot flashes, mood swings, vaginal dryness, memory loss, and sleep problems.

But there are trade-offs to consider as well. First, many women experience unwanted side effects, such as menstrual-like bleeding, water retention, breast tenderness, cramps, headaches, and problems with mood. Even more troubling is an elevated risk of breast cancer with long-term use (i.e., greater than five years), especially for those with a family history of the disease.

Side effects and concerns about breast cancer keep many women from using or continuing HRT or ERT. A 1999 national survey estimated that 37 percent of women age 50 to 74 currently take these medications. I believe that twice this many women could benefit from it. I'm also concerned that so many women miss out by dropping the treatment—fewer than 20 percent continue for at least five years. One reason may be that some important benefits are not visible. Naturally, most of us don't think about the fractures or heart attacks we *don't* suffer. As bone density testing becomes more common, I hope more women will be persuaded about the benefits of estrogen.

Birth control pills and bone

Birth control pills are prescribed for more than contraception. In premenopausal women they can correct irregular or absent menstrual cycles—problems associated with bone loss.

A recent Swedish study showed that birth control pills taken for contraception can benefit bone. Researchers interviewed two groups of women age 50 to 81. One group had experienced a hip fracture; the other group had not. Women who had used estrogen-based birth control pills in their young adult years were 25 percent less likely to have had a hip fracture. The difference was even more striking for women who'd taken birth control pills with high doses of estrogen: their risk for hip fracture was 44 percent lower.

Note: Women who use progesterone-only contraceptive measures—such as Depo-provera injections or Norplant implants—actually have bone density about 10 percent lower than average. This is a particular concern for women under age 25, who should still be gaining bone.

Deciding about hormones

Most experts—as well as national health organizations such as the American Heart Association and the National Osteoporosis Foundation—believe that most postmenopausal women would benefit from HRT or ERT. This wasn't my view as recently as five years ago, but accumulated research has become so compelling that I now agree. However, it isn't right for everyone. Hormone or estrogen replacement therapy always involves risks and benefits, and the balance is different for each individual. That's why it's so important to discuss your family and personal medical history with your doctor, and to weigh the advantages and disadvantages for yourself.

Current research suggests that taking estrogen increases breast cancer risk, while decreasing the risk of heart disease and osteoporosis. Most women fear breast cancer—and for good reason: one woman in eight will develop breast cancer in her lifetime, and the disease kills 43,000 women per year in the

United States. But surprisingly few women realize that the numbers for osteoporosis and heart disease are even more frightening.

Heart disease eventually strikes nearly *half* of all women—the toll is
233,000 women per year. And nearly 65,000 women die each year as a
consequence of osteoporosis-related hip fractures. Of course, depending on
your history, your own relative risk of breast cancer, heart disease, and osteoporosis may be quite different. Here are guidelines to discuss with your
doctor:

For women entering menopause

I believe that any woman entering menopause should consider HRT or
ERT—unless there's a contraindication: high risk for breast, uterine, or endometrial cancer; abnormal uterine bleeding of an unknown cause; a history
of blood-clotting disorders; or liver disease. Since smoking increases these
risks, it's very important for women to stop smoking if they want to take estrogen.

Factors strongly in favor include: low bone density or especially strong
risk for osteoporosis, high risk for heart disease, or debilitating menopausal
symptoms. Most professionals believe that HRT works best for bone if
started at the time of menopause and continued for at least ten years.

For women past menopause

If you're past menopause and not taking HRT or ERT, I encourage you to re-
assess this decision now and in the future. Your health and risk profile may
change; certainly our knowledge will continue to advance. Research shows
that estrogen benefits the skeleton even if started more than ten years after
menopause. For instance, one major study of women age 65 and up found
that their bone density increased by an average of 5 percent after taking hormones for three years.

Maximizing benefits—and minimizing problems—
with HRT

You can do a great deal to enhance the positive effects of HRT. As you'll see,
some of the suggestions are good advice for most older women, even if
they're not using hormones.

Pill, patch, cream, or ring?

HRT and ERT come in a variety of forms. Which kind you use depends on your treatment goals and personal preferences. Sometimes a change can make HRT more effective or easier to take.

- **Pill:** This is the most common form of HRT and ERT taken to protect the bones and heart. Some women find it difficult to remember to take the pill every day. If that's a problem, ask your doctor about switching to a brand with a convenient package that provides a helpful reminder.
- **Skin patch:** This is the second-most-popular form of HRT and ERT. An adhesive square about the size of a dollar bill folded in half is placed on your hip or abdomen. It slowly releases hormones into your blood through your skin. Though patches are just as effective as pills in protecting bone, they may not provide quite as much benefit to the heart. That's because the delivery system bypasses the liver, where cholesterol is made. The patch must be changed twice a week, so a memory-jogging routine is helpful.
- **Vaginal cream, suppository, or ring:** These allow estrogen to be applied directly to the vagina. They're valuable for treating dryness, a common postmenopausal symptom. Local action means unwanted side effects are less likely; on the other hand, you can't be assured of other estrogen benefits. Note that these products do not have FDA approval for preventing or treating osteoporosis.

Take calcium and vitamin D supplements, and stay active

Good nutrition and physical exercise boost the effectiveness of hormones. Research is beginning to quantify the benefits. One example is a study by Morris Notelovitz, M.D., Ph.D., and his colleagues at the Women's Medical and Diagnostic Center in Gainesville, Florida. They recruited women whose ovaries had been removed and who had taken ERT for at least six months.

During the study they all continued to take ERT—but half of the women also began strength training. At the end of a year those who simply took ERT had maintained their bone density. However, the women who also strength-trained showed impressive gains: an 8.3 percent increase in bone density in the spine and a 4.1 percent increase in the wrist!

Have regular medical checkups

Because HRT increases your risk for breast, uterine, and endometrial cancer, it's essential to be checked carefully before you start, and to remain vigilant as you continue. Your initial exam should include: a complete medical history to rule out contraindications such as problems with blood clots; a mammogram and manual breast exam; a pelvic examination and Pap smear. Also have a baseline bone scan—that enables you and your doctor to monitor treatment. Additional tests may be done as well, depending on your family history.

Monthly breast self-examination should be part of every woman's routine, but it's even more strongly advised for those on HRT. The same is true of annual mammograms, manual breast exams, and checkups to monitor your blood pressure and overall health. Make sure all doctors who treat you are aware that you're taking HRT.

Address any side effects

Many women who take HRT experience no problems with the medication. Indeed, women often report that they feel better, sleep better, and look better. However, this is not true for everyone. Since you'll gain the most from HRT if you continue taking it for at least ten years, it's worth the effort to deal with side effects.

Talk to your doctor about any problems you experience, such as headaches, mood changes, nausea, breast tenderness, or breakthrough bleeding. You may be advised to wait it out—often side effects disappear in just a few months. For instance, periodic breakthrough bleeding typically lasts for six to nine months, then usually stops altogether, if you are on continuous progesterone. Your doctor may suggest a different formulation—another brand or form of HRT (e.g., patch instead of pill). Yet another option to discuss is a lower dose. New research suggests that half of the usual dose can provide adequate protection for bone (though possibly not for the heart) with fewer side effects. Since progesterone is the HRT component most likely to cause problems, it might help to switch from cyclical to continuous progesterone.

Does HRT cause weight gain?

Many women swear that they gain weight on HRT. But scientific research suggests otherwise. Most studies show no weight increase when women take HRT; others show small gains—but find the same gains in women the same age who are not taking hormones.

For example, a 1997 Italian study followed twenty-seven newly menopausal women for a year. They were divided into two groups at random. Half received HRT; the other half, the control group, did not. At the beginning of the study, both groups had the same average weight and body composition. After a year, both groups had gained weight— but the control group had gained significantly *more,* an average of 3.5 pounds instead of the average 1.0 pound gained by those on HRT.

In some cases, women concerned about weight gain are simply retaining fluid. Sometimes a different HRT formulation can help. More often, though, the problem isn't HRT but two age-related changes: loss of muscle mass and inactivity. The less muscle we have, the slower our metabolism and the easier it is to gain weight. Less muscle also means we're likely to be less active and therefore burn fewer calories. When a woman tells me she's gained weight on HRT, I urge her to look at other factors that may be responsible. Strength training and aerobic exercise can often correct the problem.

Consider other bone medication if you go off HRT
Once you stop HRT, you'll experience the accelerated bone loss that women normally have after menopause. Talk to your doctor about switching to alendronate or raloxifene to maintain your bone density.

◆ ◆ ◆

A test showed slight signs of osteoporosis. I don't like to take medication unless I really need to, but my mother had a hump on her back and I don't want that, either. Good posture has always been important to me. I said, "I will not be a bent-over little old lady." I took estrogen plus two Tums in the morning and two at night. I got going on exercise— I began walking around the neighborhood; I took an osteoporosis exercise class to build strength. After I had my latest bone density test, my doctor sent back a note: "Whatever you're doing, keep up the good work."

— DOROTHY, AGE 67

◆ ◆ ◆

BISPHOSPHONATES

Bisphosphonates are among the newest medications for preventing and treating osteoporosis. They bind to the osteoclasts—the cells that break down bone—and inhibit their activities. Though new to osteoporosis, bisphosphonates have been used for several decades to treat other bone disorders. So far only one bisphosphonate has received Food and Drug Administration approval for use against osteoporosis: alendronate (Fosamax). But other drugs in this category should become available in the near future. One of these, risedronate (brand name Actonel), is currently under FDA review; research finds it's effective and safe, and I expect it to be approved soon.

Numerous studies demonstrate that alendronate can increase bone density significantly. The result is a remarkable 50 percent reduction in spine and hip fractures after only three years. Benefits begin within a year, and increase in the second and third years. There are minimal improvements after that. However, long-term use probably is necessary for continuing protection of bone. Fortunately, we know from experience with other bone diseases that bisphosphonates are safe.

Who should consider alendronate?

Alendronate is a particularly valuable option for people who are unable or unwilling to take HRT. It's also helpful for preventing the rapid bone loss that occurs in those who discontinue hormones. A 1999 Spanish study followed 144 women who stopped taking HRT. Half received alendronate; a control group was given a placebo. A year later, those in the control group showed the accelerated bone loss typically experienced by women who go off HRT: they lost an average of 3.2 percent of the bone-mineral density in their spine and 1.4 percent in their hip. But those who took alendronate maintained their hipbone density and actually gained bone—2.3 percent—in their spine.

What about using alendronate with HRT? The combination has slightly more bone benefit that either alone, so some doctors prescribe both drugs for women with severe osteoporosis.

Alendronate is tolerated well by most people, provided they follow the instructions for taking it on an empty stomach. But it can have side effects, including nausea and indigestion. Because of these problems, it's not prescribed for women who have ulcers, heartburn, or other upper gastrointestinal disorders.

Maximizing benefits and minimizing side effects

To make sure alendronate is properly absorbed, take the medication on an empty stomach along with at least 6 ounces of water, and don't drink or eat anything else for at least half an hour. This also helps prevent the gastric discomfort experienced by approximately 5 percent of women who try alendronate. In most cases, problems can be avoided by the following morning routine:

- Take the medication when you first wake up in the morning and your stomach is empty.
- Wait at least half an hour before having breakfast.
- Do not lie down for at least half an hour after taking the medication; this allows gravity to combat gastric reflux and greatly reduces heartburn.

ABOUT THE SCIENCE

Alendronate reduces fractures

After preliminary research suggested that alendronate had strong potential for treating osteoporosis, scientists from eleven clinical centers joined forces to investigate further. They recruited 2,027 women ages 55 to 80 for a study called FIT (Fracture Intervention Trial). The women already had spinal fractures caused by osteoporosis, so they were at high risk for developing additional fractures. Half were selected at random to receive alendronate; the rest were given a placebo. Over the next three years they received annual bone density tests, and records were kept of any fractures.

After three years, there was a striking difference between the two groups: Those who had taken alendronate had 47 percent fewer new fractures in their spine. They also had 51 percent fewer hip fractures and 41 percent fewer wrist fractures. These benefits are nearly as potent as those seen with long-term hormone replacement therapy, but they were evident much more quickly.

The FIT study continued with another 4,432 women age 55 to 80, but this time scientists selected women who didn't have previous fractures. Those who took alendronate had 44 percent fewer spinal fractures than those who received a placebo.

Other effective bisphosphonates (including etidronate, risedronate, pamidronate, and ibandronate) are currently under evaluation for osteoporosis treatment, but haven't yet received FDA approval. These may provide an alternative for women who suffer gastric distress from alendronate.

Katie

I've taken thyroid medication for years, so I knew I was at risk. I had a bone scan in December 1997, and the results were devastating. My bone density was off the chart for my age. I was 54, but to find numbers as low as mine, you had to look at 85-year-olds. My bones were at the low end of the range for an 85-year-old woman.

I couldn't take estrogen, because when I took birth control pills with estrogen, it gave me blood clots even on a low dose. So I began taking calcium, vitamin D, and a multivitamin. I hired a personal trainer and started working out with weights. I also took Fosamax. I had a second bone test a year later—and I had a 9.9 percent increase in bone density.

SELECTIVE ESTROGEN RECEPTOR MODULATORS (SERMS)

In the late 1980s, breast cancer researchers noticed that women taking tamoxifen (brand name Nolvadex) were experiencing an unexpected positive side effect: bone preservation. Tamoxifen belongs to a family of drugs called selective estrogen receptor modulators (SERMs). They attach to estrogen receptors on various tissues, and have mild estrogenlike effects. But they don't stimulate breast tissue the way that estrogen does. For this reason, SERMs are sometimes called "weak estrogens" (they're also called "designer estrogens"). They can be taken without increased risk of breast cancer.

Tamoxifen didn't produce the same dramatic improvements in bone as alendronate and HRT, but the accidental finding encouraged scientists to look more closely at other SERMs. In 1998 the FDA approved the first SERM for preventing osteoporosis: raloxifene (brand name Evista). And in 1999 raloxifene received FDA approval for treating osteoporosis as well.

Raloxifene is an exciting medication. Increasing bone density is only one of its benefits. It also seems to lower cholesterol to some extent (though not as much as HRT)—plus, it appears to substantially reduce the risk of breast cancer. Other promising SERMs are under investigation, and should earn FDA approval within a few years.

ABOUT THE SCIENCE

Raloxifene prevents fractures— and breast cancer

The most ambitious study of raloxifene to date is the MORE study (Multiple Outcomes of Raloxifene Evaluation), which enrolled 7,705 postmenopausal women from twenty-five different countries. All the women had osteoporosis or existing spine fractures. They were divided at random into three groups. One group received a single raloxifene tablet daily; another group received two tablets; the third group was given a placebo. Scientists followed the women for three years, giving them annual bone density tests and noting any fractures.

The control group—the women who received a placebo—had a vertebral fracture rate of 10.1 percent. The rate was 6.6 percent among women getting one tablet, and just 5.4 percent in the group getting two tablets. That's a 30 to 50 percent reduction. More research is needed to determine which dose is best for the long term.

Just as dramatic was the impact on breast cancer. Over the three-year period of the MORE study, 40 participants were diagnosed with breast cancer. But the incidence was a remarkable 76 percent lower among those taking raloxifene. New studies are under way to compare the effectiveness of raloxifene against tamoxifen for preventing breast cancer. Many believe that raloxifene will prove more effective, with fewer side effects.

Who should consider raloxifene?

Because raloxifene works by attaching to estrogen receptors, it interferes with other forms of estrogen. So it can't be taken by women who are premenopausal or by those using HRT or ERT. Like estrogen, raloxifene is not appropriate for women with liver disease or a history of or risk for blood clots.

If you're postmenopausal and not eligible for HRT—or if you would prefer not to take it—I urge you to discuss raloxifene with your doctor. This is an especially valuable option for women with a family or personal history of breast cancer.

Should you give up HRT for raloxifene? Probably not. If you have established osteoporosis, HRT or alendronate would be a better bet than raloxifene, which has only two-thirds of their fracture-reducing power. Also, raloxifene doesn't provide some of the other important benefits of HRT: While it improves cholesterol profile to some extent, it's not clear if it reduces the risk of heart disease as much as HRT does. We don't yet know if raloxifene counters the risk of Alzheimer's disease. Also, raloxifene doesn't relieve hot flashes and other menopausal discomforts—in fact, hot flashes are a common side effect in women taking the drug.

A greater concern is our lack of long-term experience with raloxifene. Though there's every indication that it's safe for extended use, we won't be certain for some time. Nor do we know what happens after a woman stops taking it, though we suspect she will again start to lose bone. Yet another question concerns possible benefits of combining raloxifene and alendronate. Though some doctors prescribe both for women who have severe or established osteoporosis, we really don't know if the combination offers any advantage over taking just one or the other. Scientists are looking at all these questions now, so we should know much more about this medication in the future.

Minimizing side effects

Raloxifene appears to have only one serious side effect: blood clots. Fortunately, these occur in just 1 percent of users. More common side effects are hot flashes (occurring in about 10 percent of those who take the drug), leg cramps (7 percent), and swelling of the hands or feet (5 to 6 percent). If you experience these problems, talk to your doctor. You may be able to lower the dose, rather than stopping the medication.

While raloxifene acts like an estrogen on bone, it doesn't have estrogen-like effects on the breast or uterus. This means that if you're taking raloxifene, you can't assume the medication is responsible for any unusual breast tenderness or vaginal bleeding. If you experience those symptoms, they should be brought to your doctor's attention.

CALCITONIN

Calcitonin is a hormone produced by the thyroid gland that reduces the bone-dissolving activity of the osteoclasts. It's normally secreted in response to elevated calcium levels in the blood. Back in the late 1970s, researchers began investigating calcitonin as a treatment for Paget's disease, a rare bone disorder. Once it became clear that calcitonin could decrease osteoclast activity, the focus expanded to include osteoporosis. Calcitonin received FDA approval for osteoporosis treatment in 1985. It remains an option for those who cannot take other osteoporosis drugs.

Calcitonin improves bone density and reduces fractures, especially fractures in the spine. After one to two years of use, spinal fractures are reduced by about 30 to 50 percent and hip fractures by about 25 percent. These improvements are comparable to those obtained from raloxifene, but less than the effects of HRT and alendronate.

One important benefit is unique to calcitonin: it can relieve the pain of recent vertebral fractures. Relief takes approximately two to four weeks. For this reason, if a woman is complaining of back pain from an osteoporotic fracture in her spine, her doctor may prescribe calcitonin along with other medications.

Who should consider calcitonin?

Current research suggests that for most women, HRT and alendronate are much more effective than calcitonin for preventing and treating osteoporosis. But any woman who can't use those drugs should consider calcitonin. It's also a valuable option for women who suffer back pain due to osteoporotic fractures. Doctors sometimes add calcitonin to HRT, alendronate, or raloxifene when a woman has severe osteoporosis or if she has not responded well to just one therapy.

Calcitonin is a protein, so it can cause allergic reactions in sensitive individuals. If you have any known allergies, discuss these with your doctor before taking calcitonin.

Minimizing side effects

Calcitonin is broken down in the stomach during digestion, so it's not effective if administered orally. Until the mid-1990s, women using calcitonin had to inject themselves every other day. Now calcitonin is available via nasal spray (brand name Miacalcin), which is much easier for most women to use. The injectable form (brand names Calcimar and Miacalcin) is still used too.

Though calcitonin is safe, some women experience side effects from the spray, including nasal irritation, redness, itchiness, and nosebleeds. The best way to avoid these problems is to alternate nostrils, taking care not to spray the medication on the same side two days in a row. Less common problems are nausea, an odd taste in the mouth, or facial flushing. If you suffer from any of these, talk to your doctor about switching to injectable calcitonin or to a different bone-preserving medication. Under development in Europe is a new oral form of calcitonin that is not broken down in the stomach.

OTHER MEDICATIONS SOMETIMES USED FOR OSTEOPOROSIS

The medications described above—HRT, ERT, alendronate, raloxifene, and calcitonin—all have FDA approval for prevention or treatment of osteoporosis, or for both. Sometimes doctors prescribe the following drugs for osteoporosis. All are approved for treating other conditions, and some probably will receive approval for treating osteoporosis after more research has been done. If your doctor suggests one of them, discuss the rationale. Often they're prescribed when a patient's bones have not responded to any of the approved medications that she's able to take.

FDA-APPROVED OSTEOPOROSIS MEDICATIONS

MEDICATION	HOW USED FOR OSTEOPOROSIS	BENEFITS	DRAWBACKS
HRT/ERT	Prevention and treatment in postmenopausal women	Improves bone density and reduces fractures; currently the most effective long-term therapy for bone. Also reduces risk of heart disease, alleviates menopausal symptoms, may reduce risk of Alzheimer's disease.	Increased risk of blood clots; slightly increased risk of breast cancer. May cause break-through bleeding, water retention, and other minor side effects.
Alendronate (Fosamax)	Prevention and treatment in post-menopausal women	Improves bone density and reduces fractures as effectively as HRT.	Can cause gastrointestinal problems—gastric reflux and heart-burn. Minimize by following careful morning routine.
Raloxifene (Evista)	Prevention and treatment in postmenopausal women	Improves bone density and reduces fractures, but not quite as well as alendronate or HRT. Also significantly reduces risk of breast cancer, can reduce cholesterol slightly.	Increased risk of blood clots. Can cause hot flashes, swelling of the arms and legs.

FDA-APPROVED OSTEOPOROSIS MEDICATIONS			
MEDICATION	HOW USED FOR OSTEOPOROSIS	BENEFITS	DRAWBACKS
Calcitonin (Miacalcin, Calcimar)	Treatment in postmenopausal women	Improves bone density in the hip and especially in the spine, but not as effectively as HRT, alendronate, or raloxifene. Relieves pain of recent spinal fractures.	Can cause facial flushing and gastrointestinal distress

Parathyroid hormone

Parathyroid hormone (PTH) is produced by the parathyroid gland in the neck. PTH—along with calcitonin and vitamin D—maintains proper levels of calcium and phosphate in the blood.

Scientists used to believe that PTH simply stimulated the osteoclasts to dissolve bone. But more recent evidence suggests that PTH acts on the osteoblasts too, stimulating bone formation. This led to the hypothesis that PTH could be combined with other medications to create a net gain in bone. A small-scale study reported in *Lancet* in 1997 showed promising benefits from adding PTH to hormone replacement therapy. Seventeen post-menopausal women received the combination, while a control group was given a placebo plus HRT. Women on HRT plus placebo maintained their bone density over a three-year period. But women who received HRT plus a low dose of PTH gained a whopping 13 percent in bone density of the spine, and they had fewer spinal fractures.

Studies of premenopausal women who develop osteoporosis because of medical problems like thyroid disorders and rheumatoid arthritis also suggest that PTH can build bone. Currently, PTH is available only in the form of daily injections, which limits its appeal. But this is a very promising medication that warrants further research.

Fluoride

This mineral has well-known benefits for teeth, and may be necessary in trace amounts for proper mineralization of bone. Early treatment studies found that fluoride could stimulate new bone formation. But there was a catch: Even though bone became denser, it wasn't quite as strong as normal bone. So women treated with fluoride actually had *more* fractures.

Newer research—using a lower dose of fluoride—shows more promising results. In one study, two hundred postmenopausal women who took fluoride for four years increased their bone density in the spine by 10 percent, and had a 70 percent reduction in spinal fractures.

In the past, side effects were an additional problem with fluoride treatment. With lower doses, problems occur less frequently. But some women report abdominal pain, bleeding in the gastrointestinal tract, vomiting, diarrhea, and joint stiffness. More research is needed to explore fluoride's potential as an osteoporosis treatment, either by itself or with other medications.

Calcitriol

As you know, vitamin D plays a key role in bone health. Vitamin D takes several different forms in the body, the most potent of which is calcitriol. Calcitriol is used to treat certain rare disorders of calcium metabolism, such as hypocalcemia (low blood calcium levels). Though one well-controlled study found that calcitriol reduced osteoporotic fractures, the benefit was no greater than that seen with ordinary vitamin D supplements. A very important concern is that calcitriol can be toxic. Until there's further research demonstrating both safety and efficacy, I don't recommend taking calcitriol to prevent or treat osteoporosis.

Testosterone

Testosterone, the male sex hormone, helps protect men from osteoporosis. Since women's bodies produce small amounts of testosterone, scientists have wondered if a testosterone boost would benefit women's bones. Preliminary evidence suggests that adding testosterone to HRT or ERT might be helpful for bone. But more research is needed. Though the FDA has approved testosterone for treatment of menopausal symptoms, its use is not yet approved for osteoporosis. Also, testosterone has significant side effects, including weight gain, lowered voice, acne, facial hair, and increased body odor.

Thiazides

Thiazides—a type of diuretic—are used to treat mild-to-moderate high blood pressure. One potentially beneficial side effect is that they conserve calcium in the kidneys, so less is excreted in the urine. Women who take thiazides for long periods (more than five years) appear to have better-than-expected bone density and a reduced risk of fractures. But the effects we've seen so far aren't strong enough to make these drugs an attractive alternative to existing medications. Further research might find ways to use thiazides more effectively. Meanwhile, if you're taking medication for blood pressure anyway, ask your doctor if thiazide would be appropriate (it isn't always). Thiazides can be taken with other medications used to treat or prevent osteoporosis.

OTHER MEDICATIONS AT THE EXPERIMENTAL STAGE

All currently approved medicines work mainly by inhibiting the bone breakdown action of the osteoclasts. Such drugs are called **antiresorptives.** On the horizon are new **stimulant** medications that promise to increase activity of the bone-building osteoblasts. They will be used alone or in combination with antiresorptives, along with exercise and nutritional supplements.

Scientists also are looking at growth factors that might stimulate bone growth. Among the candidates are hormones like growth hormone, which is produced by the pituitary gland, and Insulin-like Growth Factor (IGF), which is produced by the liver and other tissues.

Certain cytokines—a type of hormone produced at or near a site it influences—also might prove to be important. One cytokine under investigation is Transforming Growth Factor-β (TGF-β), which is produced by immune cells throughout the body. TGF-β inhibits formation of osteoclasts, which reduces their bone-destroying activity. At the same time, TGF-β stimulates formation of the bone-building osteoblasts. We now think this cytokine may play a pivotal role in bone remodeling.

Currently, investigations of growth factors and cytokines are in the infant stages. Scientists are still working with cells in test tubes or with laboratory animals. But I expect that within a decade we'll see many new medications from these important efforts.

ALTERNATIVE MEDICINE: WHAT'S PROMISING, WHAT'S NOT

Health food stores offer herbs and other products that make very appealing claims. We'd all love to find new treatments for osteoporosis that are safe, effective, and readily available. Traditionally used remedies are an excellent source of ideas for scientific study. Some of our most valuable medications—including aspirin and tamoxifen—were discovered this way. Another, ipriflavone, a synthetic compound derived from soy, has shown promise as an osteoporosis treatment in well-controlled studies.

Nevertheless, I find it both frightening and puzzling that so many women reject proven drugs in favor of untested and potentially risky herbs and medications. Anecdotal reports are no substitute for scientifically conducted clinical trials. Conventional prescription and over-the-counter drugs are required to meet FDA standards of safety and efficacy; herbal medications are not. Their purity and doses are not regulated or standardized. When you swallow one of these pill or tinctures, you have no meaningful assurance that it will do what the label promises. You can't even be sure that the medication contains the ingredients listed—or that it's free of components you don't want to take. I hope you will use alternative treatments very cautiously. Be sure to tell your doctor if you're taking these or any over-the-counter drugs.

Below are alternative medications sold in health food stores and through Internet suppliers, which herbalists sometimes recommend to treat osteoporosis. I want to emphasize that none has FDA approval or is subject to FDA regulation.

Ipriflavone

Ipriflavone is a promising treatment for osteoporosis. It's a synthetic compound derived from isoflavones—phytoestrogens found in soy—and taken in pill form. Over sixty studies, mostly from Italy, Hungary, and Japan, have found that ipriflavone improves bone density in the spine and hip of postmenopausal women by 1 to 2 percent over a two- or three-year period. While ipriflavone appears to produce few side effects, we know that it interacts with estrogen receptors. So we will need to assess its effects on the uterus, breasts, heart, and other organs.

Ipriflavone is now approved for treatment of osteoporosis in Italy, Hungary, and Japan. The research will have to meet a higher standard to gain FDA approval. Meanwhile, ipriflavone is available without prescription in many health food stores and drugstores.

Herbal treatments for menopause

Asian herbalists sometimes prescribe certain herbs for osteoporosis because they are believed to have estrogenlike effects on menopausal symptoms such as hot flashes. The hope is that they might also have estrogenlike benefits for bone. Another kind of herbal treatment involves herbs that contain high amounts of various substances found naturally in bone. Below are a few examples. Keep in mind that none of these herbs have actually been scientifically tested for this purpose, so we don't know if they actually help treat or prevent osteoporosis.

Wild yam (Dioscorea villosa)

Wild yams contain the compound diosgenin, which is used to manufacture estrogen and progesterone preparations from which prescription HRT and ERT are made. Products made from wild yams—including creams, capsules, and extracts—are sold by health food stores. The labels often bear the claim that these substances can increase the body's production of estrogen and progesterone. However, there's no scientific evidence that this actually happens.

Products made from wild yam have long been used to treat menopausal symptoms. There's limited research evidence that wild yam tames hot flashes, but even this has not been well studied. However, there's no evidence that it can treat or prevent osteoporosis. Consumers should also be aware that despite their high prices, some of these creams actually contain no yam extract!

Black cohosh, Asian ginseng, and dong quai

These roots are rich in isoflavones, and have been used by Asian herbalists to treat hot flashes in menopausal women. So far there's no scientific evidence that they're effective against hot flashes or that they're helpful to bone.

Horsetail (Equisetum arvense)

This herb—sold as tea or in tinctures—is rich in silicic acid and silicates, which provide elemental silicon. Silicon contributes to formation of both cartilage and bone. However, we normally get sufficient silicon in our diet (grains are the chief source), and there's no evidence that supplements provide any benefit to bone.

TALKING TO YOUR DOCTOR ABOUT OSTEOPOROSIS

If you're concerned about your bones—and considering medication—it's important to discuss the options with your doctor. Prepare for the visit by assembling the information your doctor needs to advise you, and by writing down any questions and concerns. Here are two checklists to get you started:

What your doctor should know

- Provide a complete family and personal medical history, including chronic diseases of your grandparents, parents, and siblings, as well as your own chronic or acute medical conditions.
- Make a list of the risk factors you identified in Chapter 4. Be sure to cover present and past lifestyle issues, such as any history of eating disorders or smoking.
- Bring a complete list of all medications you take regularly—including prescription drugs, over-the-counter medications, nutritional supplements, herbal medications, and recreational drugs.

Questions to ask if your doctor recommends medication

- Should I have a bone density test? What additional tests do I need if I've lost bone?
- Should I take calcium and vitamin D supplements?
- What exercise is appropriate for me?
- What are realistic goals regarding my bone density?
- What side effects might I experience from a particular medication?
- Are there any risks?
- Are there any symptoms that should cause me to call for advice or to stop taking the medication?
- Is there anything I can do to minimize risks and side effects?
- Should I take any other medications to prevent or treat osteoporosis?
- How long will I continue taking this medication?
- When will my bones be reevaluated to assess my success?

Like most health-conscious women, I make a point to eat well and get plenty of exercise—and I try to avoid taking medication as much as possible. Until the mid-1990s, when women asked me how to prevent osteoporosis, I advised them to keep their bones strong with a combination of good nutrition, plenty of aerobic exercise, and a strength-training routine. Though I suggested that a woman consider HRT if she already had osteoporosis, I myself didn't expect to take HRT or other preventive medication when I reached menopause.

My views have changed considerably as a result of new research and new medications. Most women can benefit from medication to prevent and treat osteoporosis. If you have bone loss, I urge you not to hesitate to use appropriate medications—they really work! When I reach menopause, I plan to evaluate my options, and if I need medication I will take it.

Standing Up to Osteoporosis

The Strong Bones Workbook

◆ ◆ ◆

Y ou've learned that it takes a combination of measures to keep your bones healthy—good nutrition and exercise for everyone, along with medication for some. The next step is to pull together all this information and put it to work.

The charts on the next two pages summarize my recommendations for women at different ages and stages. Then I'll walk you through the process of developing a personal plan for strong bones.

H O W   T O   P R O T E C T   Y O U R   B O N E S   A T   A N Y   A G E

PREMENOPAUSAL WITH NO SPECIAL RISK FACTORS	PREMENOPAUSAL WITH SIGNIFICANT RISK FACTORS	PERIMENOPAUSAL
Because you're a woman, you're at risk for osteoporosis—so you need to take care of your bones from the earliest age possible. Optimizing your bone health also optimizes your overall health.	As a woman with special risk factors, you need to pay particular attention to bone health. The same measures that protect your bones are good for your general health.	You're about to enter menopause. The first five years after menopause are the time of greatest bone loss, so it's important to get ready now.
Have regular medical checkups.	Have regular medical checkups. Talk to your doctor about having a bone density test if you have a medical condition or use medications known to increase your risk for osteoporosis.	Have regular medical checkups. Have a baseline bone density test if you haven't already had one. It's time to start thinking about HRT. At your next checkup, talk to your doctor about medical strategies for maintaining your bone.

Eat at least 1000 mg of calcium a day.
Get daily sun exposure March through October.
Consume some foods that contain vitamin D.
Eat at least five fruits and vegetables a day.
Eat soy at least once a week.

Do weight-bearing aerobic exercises and strength training.
Do balance exercises and stretching.
If you are in good health, do vertical jumping.

HOW TO PROTECT YOUR BONES AT ANY AGE		
POSTMENOPAUSAL	DIAGONOSED WITH OSTEOPENIA	DIAGNOSED WITH OSTEOPOROSIS
You are at elevated risk for osteoporosis. A combination of nutrition and exercise and possibly medication will help you maintain—or even increase—your bone density.	You are at particularly elevated risk for osteoporosis. A combination of nutrition and exercise, and most likely medication too, will help you maintain—or even increase—your bone density	A combination of nutrition, exercise, and medication will help protect you from fractures and further bone loss. Fall-prevention measures are also important.
Get regular medical checkups. Discuss HRT with your doctor. Have a baseline bone density test if you haven't already, and tests thereafter as appropriate.	Get regular medical checkups, including bone density tests as appropriate. Discuss medication with your doctor. If you're premenopausal, alendronate and calcitonin may be suggested, though they're not yet FDA approved for premenopausal women; if you're postmenopausal, you have these options as well as HRT and raloxifene.	Get regular medical checkups, including bone density tests as appropriate. Medication is strongly recommended to counter bone loss. Get referrals for specialized help if osteoporosis causes pain or emotional distress.

Take calcium and vitamin D supplements.
Eat at least 1000 mg of calcium a day if you're age 50 or younger;
    1200 mg per day if you're 51 or older.
Get daily sun exposure March through October.
Consume some foods that contain vitamin D.
Eat at least five fruits and vegetables a day.
Eat soy at least once a week.

Do weight-bearing aerobic exercise, but be careful about activities
    that might put you at risk for falls—e.g., team sports, skiing.
Do strength training to build bone.
Do balance exercises and stretching to improve flexibility and balance
    and reduce falls.

THE ONE-HOUR-PER-YEAR PLAN

Iurge you to set aside one hour each year to think about your bones. Make ten copies of the form on pages 258–59, and put them in a folder. Fill out one form now, and make a date with yourself to fill out another next year. I suggest you pick a date you're sure to remember, such as your birthday. You'll assess your current situation and make plans. Here's what to do:

Measure your height

Many parents track their kids' height on the kitchen wall to see how fast they grow. We don't think to measure ourselves. But changes in height can be a valuable warning sign of osteoporosis.

Measure your height in the morning. That's the time of day you're tallest; the tug of gravity makes you up to half an inch shorter by evening.

- Take your shoes and socks off, and stand with your back to a wall. Your feet should be close together with your heels touching the wall. Stand tall, looking straight ahead.
- Have someone place a ruler or book on your head. Keeping the ruler or book level, mark the wall at the same height as the top of your head.
- Use a tape measure or yardstick to measure your height.

If you're shorter than last year by more than half an inch—or if you've lost 1½ inches from your tallest adult height—talk to your doctor. Loss of height can be a sign of osteoporosis or other disorders.

Weigh yourself

Some women keep close track of their weight; others prefer to stay away from the scale. Either way is fine, but I believe that all women benefit from weighing themselves once a year. This can alert you to unwanted increases—the sooner you discover a change, the easier it is to correct. You also need to know about slow decreases, which can be a sign of medical problems. Most people reach a peak body weight in their fifties and sixties, then slowly lose weight in their seventies, eighties, and nineties. Low body weight is a risk factor for osteoporosis, so it's important not to lose too much.

Test your balance

I encourage you to take the balance tests in Chapter 6 every year. Starting in our forties and fifties, coordination and balance usually begin to decline. If you see changes, you'll know to take steps to correct them. If you're following the exercise program in this book, you'll probably see encouraging improvements.

Assess your eating habits

Our eating patterns can change along with other changes in our lives—getting married, having children, moving, or even buying a new cookbook. So it's helpful to look at our diet periodically.

- Take the calcium quiz in Chapter 7 (page 107) to see if you're getting enough. This will help you decide if you need to change your diet or take supplements.
- Do you get enough vitamin D from food or the sun?
- Do you consume at least five servings of fruits and vegetables daily?
- Are you eating soy at least once a week?

Evaluate your physical activity

Assessing your exercise habits can help you stay on track and plan an effective fitness program for the coming year.

- How many hours do you spend each week in vigorous aerobic activity? How much of that time is spent on weight-bearing activities?
- Are you strength-training at least twice a week?
- If you're younger than 50 and in good health, have you been doing one to two minutes of vertical jumping three to six days a week?
- Do you take time for balance exercises?
- Do you stretch after every workout or at other times during the day?

Update your medical records

Include information on the following:

- Bone density testing—keep your test results in a folder
- Immunizations and routine tests, such as mammograms
- Medical conditions
- Medications taken regularly (including over-the-counter and herbal treatments)
- Significant medical conditions of your siblings and parents

Make an appointment for an annual medical checkup

Early detection of diseases, including osteoporosis, offers the best hope for successful treatment. Discuss osteoporosis with your doctor, and ask about bone density testing. Have the doctor check your spine for changes in posture.

Check your home for fall hazards

Little changes around the house can increase the risk of falling. Maybe a light burned out in a stairway, where it's slightly inconvenient to replace. Or perhaps you bought a new rug but haven't gotten around to buying a skid-proof pad to go under it.

This is a good opportunity to give your house a quick safety review. See page 95 for a check list. Correcting hazards is important for your guests as well as for you.

Think about your lifestyle

You've already thought about your food and exercise habits. What other changes would you like to make for better health?

- Do you smoke?
- Are you drinking too much—more than one drink per day?
- Are you overdoing caffeine—more than 400 milligrams (e.g., four cups of coffee) per day?
- Is there too much stress in your life?

Smoking, as well as excess consumption of alcohol or caffeine, increases your risk for osteoporosis.

List your accomplishments and goals for change

Go back over the form, and note the ways in which you're taking good care of your bones. Also jot down areas that need improvement.

Take some time to think about your goals for the coming year. What would help you succeed? What difficulties do you anticipate along the way? How can you overcome them? Later in the chapter I'll suggest how you can work with this list.

Your needs may change over time

In 1985 Marie's team placed first at the Ocean State Marathon in Newport, Rhode Island. The next day she had a bone density test and learned that she had osteoporosis. She was 51.

Marie tackled this challenge with characteristic energy. She developed a forty-five-minute morning exercise routine including sit-ups, push-ups, back exercises, and stretches. She began strength training three times a week. And as her schedule permitted, she walked, ran, swam, took a water exercise class, and cross-country-skied. In addition to exercising, Marie added calcium to her diet, and took a calcium supplement and vitamin D. Her doctor prescribed estrogen. All these efforts paid off for more than a decade: Marie's bone density increased by 5 to 6 percent.

But last year her annual bone density test revealed a decrease. Another warning sign was a broken toe. At her doctor's suggestion, Marie has begun taking Fosamax, as well as continuing the other measures. Says Marie, "I'm hoping for better test results next year."

THE *STRONG WOMEN, STRONG BONES*
ONE-HOUR SELF-ASSESSMENT CHECKLIST

Date ——————

Height (measured in the morning)

——————

Weight (measured in the morning)

——————

Balance test score

——————

☐   Completed home safety checkup

Corrections needed

————————————————

————————————————

Nutrition

Approximate daily calcium intake (mg): ——————

Do I need a calcium supplement?   ☐ Yes   ☐ No

Do I need extra vitamin D?   ☐ Yes   ☐ No

Do I consume a total of at least five fruits and vegetables
   per day?   ☐ Yes   ☐ No

Do I eat at least one serving of soy per week?   ☐ Yes   ☐ No

Exercise

Weight-bearing aerobic exercise:

Average number of sessions per week: ——— Average minutes/session: ———

Types of weight-bearing exercise: ————————————————————

Strength training:

Average number of sessions per week: ———

Heaviest ankle weight used: ——— lbs. Heaviest dumbbell used: ——— lbs

Do I do vertical jumping (for premenopausal women)?   ☐ Yes   ☐ No

Do I do balance training every week?   ☐ Yes   ☐ No

Do I stretch after each workout?   ☐ Yes   ☐ No

THE *STRONG WOMEN, STRONG BONES* ONE-HOUR SELF-ASSESSMENT CHECKLIST

Medical appointments

☐ Annual checkup
☐ Bone density test (if needed)

Tests taken this year

_____

_____

Immunizations received this year

_____

Medical Updates

Self

_____

_____

_____

_____

Siblings and parents

_____

_____

_____

Lifestyle concerns

(check all that apply)

☐ Smoking
☐ Alcohol
☐ Caffeine
☐ Stress

Accomplishments

Exercise _____

_____

Nutrition _____

_____

Medical _____

_____

Lifestyle _____

_____

Goals

Exercise _____

Nutrition _____

Medical _____

Lifestyle _____

HOW TO GET STARTED

As you read this book, you may have decided to change your diet, to start taking nutritional supplements, to begin several different kinds of physical exercise, to quit smoking, to cut back on caffeine and alcohol, to schedule a medical checkup, and to have a bone density test. Whew!

Some people meet such challenges very easily. But most of us find it difficult to face numerous tasks, some of which involve several components. We feel overwhelmed; we procrastinate. In my experience—and there's research to back me up—there are two simple secrets to success:

Plan

Complete the one-hour assessment on pages 258–59. Then set aside another half hour to make plans. Sit down with this book, your calendar, and a pad and pencil, and go back over the form you filled out.

Do you want to make changes in your diet? Make a shopping list (see page 261). Have you decided to take calcium supplements? Figure out which kind, and decide when you're going to take them during the day.

What about exercise? Do you need to buy equipment? Make a list, and order by mail. Or check the Yellow Pages and put a shopping appointment on your calendar. Figure out which days and what times you plan to exercise, and add those appointments to your calendar too.

If you're due for a medical checkup, call your doctor.

Think about your goals—and any obstacles you anticipate. What will it take to make them happen?

B O N E - F R I E N D L Y   S H O P P I N G   L I S T

DAIRY

- ☐ milk
- ☐ buttermilk
- ☐ yogurt
- ☐ cottage cheese
- ☐ ricotta
- ☐ cheddar, Swiss, Parmesan cheese
- ☐ protein-fortified cream cheese
- ☐ frozen yogurt

SOY PRODUCTS AND BEANS

- ☐ soy milk
- ☐ calcium-fortified soy beverage
- ☐ soybeans, soy nuts
- ☐ tofu made with calcium sulfate
- ☐ tempeh
- ☐ textured vegetable protein
- ☐ miso paste
- ☐ beans—dry, canned (kidney, navy, chick-peas, pinto)

FRESH FISH

- ☐ ocean fish
- ☐ trout, bass
- ☐ clams, oysters, lobster, shrimp

VEGETABLES

- ☐ spinach
- ☐ kale
- ☐ mustard greens
- ☐ collard greens
- ☐ lettuce
- ☐ green beans
- ☐ broccoli
- ☐ cauliflower
- ☐ potatoes
- ☐ squash
- ☐ sweet potatoes
- ☐ celery
- ☐ onions
- ☐ carrots
- ☐ mushrooms
- ☐ peas
- ☐ eggplant
- ☐ brussels sprouts
- ☐ cabbage
- ☐ peppers
- ☐ cucumbers
- ☐ tomatoes
- ☐ radishes
- ☐ scallions
- ☐ dill, parsley
- ☐ basil, other herbs
- ☐ garlic
- ☐ special in-season vegetables
- ☐ canned tomatoes
- ☐ tomato sauce
- ☐ vegetable juice

FRUITS AND JUICES

- ☐ calcium-fortified orange juice
- ☐ oranges
- ☐ grapefruits
- ☐ lemons, limes
- ☐ tangerines
- ☐ mango
- ☐ rhubarb
- ☐ kiwi
- ☐ raisins
- ☐ prunes (dried)
- ☐ apples
- ☐ pears
- ☐ peaches
- ☐ plums
- ☐ bananas
- ☐ melon
- ☐ pineapple
- ☐ strawberries
- ☐ blueberries
- ☐ dried fruit
- ☐ special in-season fruit

OTHER GROCERIES

- ☐ calcium-enriched cold cereal
- ☐ canned fish (salmon, anchovies, sardines, tuna)
- ☐ nuts (almonds, hazelnuts)
- ☐ dry nonfat milk

Keep logs

Filling out an exercise or nutrition log takes just a few seconds. But research consistently shows that this is the single most effective way to ensure success. Make copies of the logs on pages 263 and 264, and put them in a folder.

Nutrition logs

I suggest that you post each week's food log on your refrigerator or in some other handy place. Use it daily for at least a few weeks. After that, you might not need it—but I encourage you to use it once a month to make sure you're still eating all the foods you need for healthy bones.

Exercise logs

The exercise program in this book involves five separate components; within one of these components—strength training—there are ten different exercises. You'll make progress from week to week, and will need to adjust the length of your aerobic workouts and the amount of weight you lift. That's a lot to keep track of! Written logs make your exercise sessions more efficient. And it's so satisfying to look back a few months from now and see how far you've come.

◆ ◆ ◆

Some of my friends get their exercise from recreation. Exercise is like a vitamin pill to me. I have to go into that room on a prescribed day and do it for a prescribed time. I keep written records.

— PAM

◆ ◆ ◆

STRONG WOMEN, STRONG BONES
Food Log

	GOAL	SUN	MON	TUES	WED	THU	FRI	SAT
Calcium Per serving ✓✓✓ = excellent source ✓✓ = good source ✓ = minor source	Up to age 50: At least 10 ✓ /day Age 50 and up: At least 12 ✓ /day							
Vitamin D ✓ = 10–15 minutes of sun ✓ = 1 serving vitamin D–rich food ✓✓ = 400 IU supplement	Up to age 50: 1 ✓ /day Age 50–70: 2 ✓ /day Age 70 and up: 3 ✓ /day							
Fruits and vegetables ✓ = 1 serving	At least 5/day							
Soy foods ✓ = 1 serving	At least 1/week							

✓✓✓ = EXCELLENT CALCIUM SOURCE
   milk, yogurt, ricotta, cheddar, Swiss, soy milk and calcium-fortified soy beverages, tofu made with calcium sulfate, soy nuts, salmon canned with bones, calcium-fortified orange juice and calcium-fortified breakfast cereal
✓✓ = GOOD CALCIUM SOURCE
   soft cheese, ice cream, frozen yogurt, soybeans, rhubarb, sardines, anchovies
✓ = MINOR CALCIUM SOURCE
   cottage cheese, cream cheese, and other soft cheese, beans, almonds, hazelnuts, leafy greens, broccoli, green beans, squash, fresh fish and seafood, prunes, raisins, oranges, tangerines, grapefruit, mango, kiwi
✓ = VITAMIN D–RICH FOOD

STRONG WOMEN, STRONG BONES
Exercise Log

EXERCISE	GOAL (fill in)	SUN	MON	Tues	WED	THU	FRI	SAT
Aerobic activity (minutes)								
Vertical jumping (✓ if appropriate)	3–6 days/ week							
Strength training (8 reps × 2 sets)	3 times/ week	Fill in pounds or level for each session						
Squat or lunge								
Step up								
Overhead press								
Forward fly								
Back extension								
Abdominal								
Side leg raise								
Ankle exercise								
Chest press								
Biceps curl								
Balance exercises Mountain pose One-legged stork Tandem walk	3–6 days/ week							
Stretches Hamstring Shoulder Upper back	After each workout							

◆ ◆ ◆

For a week or so after the diagnosis I was really upset about it. But you have to buckle down and do something. I got my test results on January 21, and on January 23 I started doing the exercises. I work out three or four times a week. I stay motivated because I don't want to be crippled. I have no problem at all staying motivated.

—ANN

◆ ◆ ◆

DEALING WITH TEMPORARY SETBACKS

It's not easy to establish new habits! Making significant changes in your eating and exercise patterns takes time. If you persist, it will happen. Try to be patient with yourself.

If you're having trouble getting started

This is an ambitious program. Though I've tried to make it doable, you might need a more gradual start. For instance, instead of adopting the full nutrition program, you could begin by adding one fruit or vegetable serving per day. You could start with just the aerobic portion of the exercise program, and do only ten minutes of exercise three times a week. Set yourself a goal you're sure you can achieve, then build upon your success. What's important for strong bones is consistency over a long period of time. It doesn't matter if it takes you a little longer to get there.

If you've gone off track

Nobody is perfect. I know I'm not. Even though I love to eat good wholesome food and I love to exercise, I occasionally have periods when my lifestyle isn't what I want it to be—if I get sick, if I'm traveling and on a tight schedule, if pressing family needs interfere. What's important is that I make sure these periods are as brief as possible. A few tips:

Need a motivation boost?

• **Write down your goals**
Focusing on what you want to achieve, and seeing the list on paper, can be magical.

• **Add some variety**
Routines are great for regularity, but the same-old, same-old can get boring. Buy a cookbook and try some new recipes. Swap exercises, change your walking route, or buy some new tapes if you listen to a personal stereo as you work out.

• **Recruit a partner**
Having a diet or workout buddy is a proven motivator. Exercise dates are a terrific way to socialize with friends and family.

• **Join a club or class**
Get variety and companionship all at once. Community centers and adult education programs are often very inexpensive.

• **Do *something*.** Don't think of lifestyle changes as an all-or-nothing proposition. It's much better—both for your body and for maintaining good habits and motivation—to do a little bit rather than to do nothing. Focus on having one nutritious meal (even if the others are less than ideal). Take a short walk, or do the wide leg squats even if you can't get through the entire exercise program.
• **Get back on track as soon as possible.** If it seems overwhelming, start small and build up gradually.
• **Don't feel guilty!** Figure out why you went astray, and think how you might avoid the problem in the future. Then congratulate yourself and move on.

WHEN EXERCISE HURTS

Exercise should make you feel great. True, you might experience brief discomfort, especially at the beginning. If you've been sedentary, your muscles might feel a little sore during the first few weeks. And when you're strength training at level 4, you feel muscle fatigue during the last few lifts. But the exercises described in this book should never cause acute pain.

How it feels	What it means	What to do
Dull ache in the muscles that increases during a workout, but disappears as soon as you stop.	Normal muscle fatigue	If the ache is unpleasant, use a slighly lighter weight.
Muscle soreness the day after a workout.	Delayed muscle soreness is normal. It should disappear in a few days.	Try stretching. Hot baths or massage can help.
Sharp pain in your back or a joint that doesn't go away quickly.	You may have uncovered a preexisting injury or injured yourself.	Stop the exercise. Rest the affected area, and treat it with ice. Resume the activity in few days at lower intensity—if you're strength training, use lighter weights and a more limited range of motion; slow down if it's aerobic exercise. If pain persists or gets worse, consult your doctor.
Chest pain or tightness during aerobic exercise; severe shortness of breath.	These symptoms could indicate cardiac problems.	Stop your workout immediately and call your doctor.

If you need individual help

Working one-on-one with a professional can be enormously helpful, especially if you have special needs or if you're finding it hard to get started. This kind of assistance may not be as expensive as you'd think. HMOs and insurance plans may cover classes or individual consultations, especially if you've been diagnosed with osteoporosis. If you belong to a health club or community center, ask what resources are available there. Also check to see if there are relevant adult education classes available in your area.

Four kinds of specialists that I often recommend are:

Nutritionist

A registered dietitian can assist if you're having trouble changing your diet to include more calcium, vitamin D, fruits, and vegetables. The initials R.D., which stand for registered dietician, mean that a nutritionist has met the stringent requirements of the American Dietetic Association. To find an R.D. in your area, talk to your doctor or contact the American Dietetic Association at 1-800-366-1655 or http://www.eatright.org.

Personal trainer

Personal trainers aren't just for movie stars! Even if you can't afford to have someone coach you through every workout, it's often very useful to schedule one or two sessions with a trainer when you're starting a program and learning the moves, or if you want to change your routine. A trainer can be particularly valuable if you have special physical needs or limitations, and need to adapt the exercises.

Your doctor may be able to recommend a trainer. Or you could get a referral from a local health club (even if you're not a member) or adult education program. If you have special medical concerns, such as osteoporosis, make sure the trainer has experience working with people like you. The trainer should have certification from at least one of the following organizations: the American College of Sports Medicine, the National Strength and Conditioning Association, the National Academy of Sports Medicine, the American Council on Exercise, Aerobics and Fitness Association of America,

IDEA (the International Association of Fitness Professionals), or the Cooper Institute for Aerobics Research.

◆ ◆ ◆

I'm at the point now where if I don't exercise I feel annoyed. It's something I really need to do. Afterwards, I feel better about everything in general.

— LIZ

◆ ◆ ◆

Psychotherapist

Learning that you have osteopenia or osteoporosis can be frightening; it can affect your self-image and self-confidence. Wendi said:

> "I'm 48 years old and was diagnosed with osteoporosis earlier this year. I wasn't expecting it—I've always been an avid exerciser. The news was devastating. I haven't told many people about it. Probably no one would expect it from me, because I'm the most active, healthy-looking person in my whole group of friends and co-workers. I felt almost marred. Over the past months, I've experienced some signs of clinical depression. I'm currently getting help to find out why."

Many women become depressed, anxious, angry, or fearful after their diagnosis. If strong negative reactions linger for more than a few weeks, or if you sense that emotional issues are interfering with your ability to make necessary changes in your diet or physical activity, I urge you to talk to a mental health professional. A few sessions with a trained therapist can help you sort out and deal with these feelings. Good referral sources are your doctor, or the psychology or psychiatry department at a local teaching hospital.

Physical therapist

Bone fractures often cause pain or physical limitations. A physical therapist can alleviate these problems with special exercises to improve your strength and flexibility. The therapist also can help you modify the program in this book so that you get the most out of it. If you think you'd benefit from this kind of assistance, ask your doctor to refer you to a licensed physical therapist. Your medical insurance may cover this treatment—check to be sure.

You're starting a program that will change your life. You'll do everything possible to protect your bones and avoid the devastating fractures that cripple so many women each year. But the results of this program go beyond your bones. Eating well and being physically active also promote overall health and well-being. You'll probably enjoy more energy during the day and sleep better at night. Gaining physical strength is empowering emotionally as well. And you can take tremendous satisfaction in what you're accomplishing for yourself. I've worked with many women who've made these changes. They tell me that they feel so good, they can't imagine living any other way. I wish you the same joy and success as you begin.

Men Get Osteoporosis Too!

◆ ◆ ◆

A man's wife e-mailed me recently. Her husband was told by his physician, "Men don't get osteoporosis." It's like women being told for so many years that cardiovascular disease is solely a problem of men.

—Jerome C. Donnelly
Men's Osteoporosis Online Support Group
http://pages.prodigy.net/jerryd3001/

Most men are astonished to learn that they too can lose bone and suffer fractures. In fact, it's a common problem. An estimated two million American men have osteoporosis, and another three million have osteopenia. Each year, 100,000 men fracture a hip. Over a lifetime, about one man in five will suffer an osteoporotic fracture—more than will develop prostate cancer.

Despite these alarming numbers, male osteoporosis often goes undiagnosed because men—and even doctors—think of it as a women's disease. In a recent Gallup survey, fewer than 2 percent of men had been warned by their doctor that they might be at risk for osteoporosis.

◆ ◆ ◆

I had to switch doctors, and got a lady doctor. She asked about my back; she looked at my records—and she suggested I have a bone density test. She said that because of my posture, my history of backaches, and the fact

that I was shrinking in height, I might have osteoporosis. She was right.
I'm lucky I saw a woman doctor, because she was more in tune with it.

I was 53 and in good health. I'd been going in for an annual physical with
a male doctor for seven or eight years, and he never said anything. A few
years ago I donated a kidney to my brother, and I went through a lot of
testing, but nothing showed up. I didn't know men got osteoporosis—I
thought osteoporosis was old ladies all bent over.

—DICK

◆ ◆ ◆

Men have more time to protect themselves than women do. Typically they start out with stronger bones. Though they lose bone mass as they get older, they don't experience the sudden drop that women have at menopause. So it takes longer for men to reach the danger point. But if they live long enough, they too are at risk for fractures.

Much of the information in this book applies to men as well as women. The same preventive measures—good nutrition and physical activity—help men too. Men can take the same bone density tests. Medication can be helpful for them as well, though different drugs may be prescribed for men. This chapter explains how men can benefit from the *Strong Women, Strong Bones* program.

HOW MEN'S BONES DEVELOP

On average, men have 25 percent more bone mass than women do. One reason is testosterone, the male sex hormone, which stimulates bone and muscle growth. Also, men tend to be more physically active than women, and that helps build muscle too. Diet plays a part as well. Because men are larger, more muscular, and more active, they generally eat more than we do. So they typically get more calcium and other nutrients.

Like women, men start to lose bone in their late thirties or early forties. But the process is much slower for them. Instead of losing .5 to 1 percent of their bone each year, as typically happens to women in those years, men lose only about .3 percent annually. Changes remain slow as a man enters his fifties, in contrast to the accelerated bone loss of a woman after menopause. As I explained in Chapter 2, women lose bone mainly because osteoclast activity increases, and too much bone is broken down. With men, the mechanism is different: bone loss usually occurs because less bone is formed.

Men also lose strength and balancing ability as they get older, which increases their risk of falls. Beginning around age 30, men lose about 1 percent of their muscle strength each year. The change accelerates to about 2 percent per year after age 60. By the time a man reaches 80, typically he's lost about 60 percent of the strength he had at age 30.

Women begin to have osteoporotic fractures in their fifties. Men—thanks to higher peak bone mass and slower bone loss—usually have another decade or two before they reach the danger zone.

Symptoms of osteoporosis

If you've experienced any of these symptoms, you might have osteopenia or osteoporosis. Discuss this possibility with your doctor and ask about bone density testing. The earlier you know, the sooner you can take preventive measures.

• Fractures caused by slight to moderate trauma
• Loss of height of more than an inch and a half
• Curvature of the spine or hunched-over posture
• Chronic back pain, usually in the middle or upper back

◆ ◆ ◆

I used to be almost 5 feet 11 inches. Now I'm 5 feet 7¼ inches. A woman in my office has osteoporosis. We talked about it, and about the fact that I was shrinking. My name is Dick and one of the gals at work gave me a nickname: the Incredible Shrinking Dick.

◆ ◆ ◆

MEN AT RISK

All men past age 65—like women age 50 and up—should consider themselves at risk for osteoporosis. But some younger men are at risk too. Except for hormone-related issues, risk factors are the same for men as they are for women. Discuss bone density testing with your doctor if any of the following apply:

Low testosterone levels

Hormonal stimulation is just as important for men's bones as it is for women's. Low testosterone levels are responsible for about half the cases of osteoporosis in men. Usually, low testosterone is a consequence of aging. But certain medical conditions can lead to more rapid loss. Signs of low testosterone include the following:

- Reduced libido or impotence
- Decreased facial and body hair
- Enlarged breasts

If you experience these changes, discuss them with your doctor so the cause can be determined and addressed. Many men have low testosterone levels without any symptoms at all. A blood test can measure testosterone levels. If you're diagnosed with low testosterone, your doctor might suggest a bone density test in addition to other diagnostic tests and treatments.

Racial heritage and family history

With men as with women, fair skin is associated with higher risk of osteoporosis. Black and Hispanic men can get osteoporosis, but it generally happens even later than it does for other men.

If close relatives—your parents or siblings—have experienced bone loss or fractures, you're at higher risk. The reason could be genetic, or it could be related to diet and lifestyle patterns acquired from your family.

Body type

Men with a light frame and low body weight have a higher risk of osteoporosis. Consider yourself at elevated risk if your BMI is lower than 19 (see table on page 55).

Dieting and eating disorders

We associate eating disorders with young women, but surprising numbers of young men—especially competitive athletes in sports with weight classifications—suffer from the problem. If you've been a yo-yo dieter, or if you've had anorexia or bulimia, you're at higher risk for bone loss.

Medical history and medications

Men are affected by the same medical conditions and medications that put women at higher risk (see pages 56–61 for more detail):

Conditions	Medications
Rheumatoid arthritis	Steroids
Diseases of the thyroid or parathyroid	Anticonvulsants
Diabetes Type 1	Diuretics other than thiazide
Lactose intolerance	Antacids containing aluminum
Other chronic digestive disorders	

Lifestyle

The following increase risk of osteoporosis for men as well as women (see pages 61–63 for further information):

- Inactivity
- Diet low in calcium and vitamin D
- High alcohol consumption
- Smoking (current or past)

TESTING RECOMMENDATIONS FOR MEN

National health organizations, such as the National Osteoporosis Foundation, have developed bone density–testing guidelines for women. But so far, there are no such guidelines for men. I expect this omission will be corrected as the baby boomers age and male osteoporosis becomes a more visible problem.

The earlier bone loss is diagnosed, the easier it is to treat. Discuss bone density testing with your doctor if any of the following apply to you:

- You have low testosterone levels.
- You have symptoms of osteopenia or osteoporosis, including fractures, curvature of the spine, loss of height, or chronic back pain.
- You have a medical condition that causes bone loss.
- You take a medication that causes bone loss.
- You're about to start treatment for bone loss.

Though bone density tests are performed in the same way for men and women, the results are interpreted differently. Instead of comparing men to young women to calculate T-scores, comparisons are made to young men.

◆ ◆ ◆

I took all kinds of tests, and they said I have idiopathic osteoporosis. I asked, "What does that mean in my language?" The doctor said, "You're ten times more likely to break a bone than someone else your age. And we don't know why."

—DICK

◆ ◆ ◆

ADAPTING THE *STRONG WOMEN, STRONG BONES* PROGRAM FOR MEN

For men, as for women, osteoporosis prevention and treatment rest on the three foundations of nutrition, exercise, and medication. But some of the specifics are different. Here's how men should modify the *SWSB* program:

Nutrition

The same nutrients that are important for women's bones are helpful for men too. Because men are larger and eat more, they usually consume more of these essential nutrients—calcium, vitamin D, magnesium, vitamin K, vitamin C, and potassium. Nevertheless, a man who has osteopenia or osteoporosis should take a calcium and vitamin D supplement, following the guidelines in Chapter 7 (pages 112–14). Research described earlier (page 116) found a significant reduction in fractures for older men as well as women who took 500 milligrams per day of calcium and 700 IU per day of vitamin D.

Exercise

We suspect that men's bones react to exercise in the same positive way that women's bones do, but we don't yet have detailed research confirmation. However, we know enough about the other health benefits of exercise to feel confident about recommending it.

Weight-bearing aerobic exercise
Men can follow the same program that women use.

High-impact exercise
Men age 50 and under who are in good health can do the vertical jumps, following the instructions for women.

Strength training

Because men, on average, are stronger than women, most can start with slightly heavier weights. Men usually reach levels that are 25 to 50 percent higher than those reached by women the same age. Otherwise, the instructions are the same for men and women.

Here's how to adapt the *SWSB* strength-training program in this book if you're a man:

- Instead of starting with 3- and 5-pound weights, begin with 5- and 8-pound dumbbells. However, don't hesitate to use lighter weights if you prefer—you will progress as you get stronger.
- Use the table to set goals. They're meant to be upper limits—you may advance even farther. But heed the same caution I give women: Don't go above 20 pounds with the ankle weights or above 25 pounds with dumbbells, since heavier versions could become a problem for your joints.

Balance exercises and stretching

Men can follow the same program that women use.

Medication

Currently, there are no medications with FDA approval for preventing or treating osteoporosis in men. There is an urgent need for research in this area. Meanwhile, physicians treat men with some of the same medications they use for women.

The first medication considered for men with low bone density is testosterone replacement therapy. But this is used only if a man has low levels of testosterone. Other medications prescribed for men include:

Bisphosphonates (Fosamax)

Recent studies indicate that Fosamax is effective for men as well as women. Many physicians are already using it to treat male patients with osteoporosis, and FDA approval is expected soon. Other bisphosphonates under development may eventually gain approval for use in men as well.

STRENGTH-TRAINING GOALS FOR MEN			
EXERCISE	20 TO 49 YEARS OLD	50 TO 69 YEARS OLD	70 YEARS AND OLDER
Wide leg squat	Work toward not touching the chair and add 8- to 12-pound dumbbells	Work toward not touching the chair and add 5- to 10-pound dumbbells	Work toward not touching the chair and add 3- to 8-pound dumbbells
Step up	Two steps, with 8- to 12-pound dumbbells	Two steps, with 5- to 10-pound dumbbells	Two steps with 3- to 8-pound dumbbells
Seated overhead press	10 to 20 pounds	8 to 18 pounds	5 to 15 pounds
Forward fly	12 to 15 pounds	8 to 12 pounds	5 to 8 pounds
Back extension	In good form	In good form	In good form
Abdominal exercise	Reverse curl	Reverse curl	Reverse curl
Side leg raise	12 to 18 pounds	8 to 15 pounds	5 to 12 pounds
Ankle exercise	Push and pull toes with 15- to 20-pound ankle weights	Push and pull toes with 10- to 15-pound ankle weights	Push and pull toes with 8- to 12-pound ankle weights
Chest press	15 to 25 pounds	12 to 20 pounds	8 to 18 pounds
Biceps curl with rotation	20 to 25 pounds	12 to 20 pounds	10 to 15 pounds
Front lunge	Controlled and with good balance, using 10- to 15-pound dumbbells	Controlled and with good balance, using 8- to 12-pound dumbbells	Controlled and with good balance, using 5- to 8-pound dumbbells
Wrist curl	6 to 10 pounds	5 to 8 pounds	3 to 5 pounds

Calcitonin (Miacalcin or Calcimar)

This medication seems to work for men, though we don't yet have enough research evidence to support FDA approval.

Parathyroid hormone and fluoride

Neither of these drugs is approved for women or for men, but they're sometimes used for men who can't be successfully treated by other medications.

Osteoporosis can catch men unawares. But the consequences of this disease are just as devastating for men as they are for women. So prevention and early detection are every bit as important.

Jerry

Iwas 50, and I'd been having back pain for fifteen years. The pain was aggravated by my work as a dentist. I was referred to a major medical center. They took one look at my X rays and said, "You have compression fractures in your spine and you probably have osteoporosis." They did a DXA and I was −2.5 standard deviations in the spine.

When I found out I had osteoporosis, you could have knocked me over with a feather. I didn't know that men got osteoporosis. I've always had a healthy diet, and exercise was a big part of my life. Tests showed hypogonadism—low testosterone. Also, years earlier, when I was in dental school, I was treated for allergies with steroid injections. This might be involved too.

I take testosterone, Fosamax, and a calcium supplement with vitamin D. I still exercise, and I'm doing strength training now too. I eat lots of fruits and vegetables. My most recent bone density tests showed a 21 percent improvement in my spine in the five years since my diagnosis. My spine is now in the low-normal range—I wouldn't even be considered osteopenic now. The backache is much better. I count my blessings. If this had happened ten years ago I would have been crippled by now. Fosamax is a wonder drug as far as I'm concerned.

CHAPTER 12

Questions and Answers

◆ ◆ ◆

A s I wrote this book, I tried to anticipate your concerns. But you may still have questions. I hope you'll find the answers in this chapter. If not, please check the index—it's so easy to miss a detail as you read the book.

OSTEOPOROSIS

Q: *My spine is bent forward from osteoporosis. Is it possible to regain my youthful posture?*

A: The characteristic bent-over posture of osteoporosis is caused by fractures in the spine. Unfortunately, broken vertebras can't regain their original shape. However, if you strengthen the muscles of your shoulders and upper back, your posture can improve. Exercise, along with medication and good nutrition, will help prevent further deterioration.

Q: *I had scoliosis as a child—does this make me more vulnerable to osteoporosis?*

A: We suspect that it might. Scientists are researching this question because we know that many women who develop osteoporosis also have scoliosis, or curvature of the spine. Because of this association, I suggest you talk to your doctor about having a bone density test.

Q: *I broke my lower leg recently as the result of a simple fall. Is it possible to have osteoporosis in bones other than the hip, spine, and wrist?*

A: Osteoporosis affects the entire skeleton, though fractures most commonly occur in the bones of the spine, hip and wrist. If you break *any* bone from a minor fall, talk to your doctor about having a bone density test.

Q: *I have osteoarthritis. Someone told me that this makes me immune to osteoporosis. Is that true?*

A: Individuals with osteoarthritis—a condition in which joint cartilage degenerates—are not immune to osteoporosis. However, they do appear to have lower risk for bone loss. We're not sure why this is true, but one reason could be that people who get osteoarthritis tend to be heavier. Overweight is hard on the joints, but it protects against osteoporosis.

Q: *My mom, who's 82, has lost height and is bent over. Does this mean she has osteoporosis?*

A: Given her age and symptoms, it's is a strong possibility. But the only way she can be sure is to have a bone density test. Since she has curvature of the spine, she should also have a spine X ray to check for fractures.

BONE DENSITY TESTING

Q: *They redid my DXA scan, making me lie on my side. How come?*

A: A DXA test picks up all bone mineral in the scanned area. Sometimes this includes calcium deposits in arteries and calcifications around the spine, which aren't related to bone density. Some scanners can take a side view of the spine that allows the technician to correct for irrelevant calcium. Otherwise, you'll need to lie on your side.

Q: *My doctor just installed a DXA in her office, and she's recommended that I have a bone scan. I'm 30 years old and in good health. Does this sound right?*

A: A 30-year-old woman with no special risk factors for osteoporosis probably does not need a DXA test. Ask your doctor why she is making this recommendation. While testing wouldn't be harmful, you'd probably have to pay for it—your insurance company is unlikely to pick up the tab unless you're at risk. Unfortunately, some physicians overprescribe bone density tests after they invest in expensive DXA equipment.

Should I be concerned about radiation exposure when I have a bone density test?

Excessive radiation exposure can cause cancer and other serious medical problems. Fortunately, bone density can be tested with only minimal radiation—so little that the technician can safely remain in the room.

All of us are exposed to radiation from environmental sources (including the sun and the ground we live on); most adults also have some exposure from medical procedures. Radiation exposure is usually measured in millirems, or mrems. Here are a few examples:

Radiation source	Approximate exposure (in mrem)
Environment (in the United States)	0.5–1.5 per day
SXA (single X-ray absorptiometry)	1–2
DXA (dual X-ray absorptiometry)	1–3
RA (radiographic absorptiometry)	5
Coast-to-coast flight	5
Standard chest X ray	25
Full dental X ray	200–300

NUTRITION

Q: *Can I use a tanning lamp to get more vitamin D?*

A: You could use a tanning lamp as a source of vitamin D, because the special lightbulb triggers the same reaction in your skin as the sun does. However, tanning lamps, like the sun, carry a risk of skin cancer, which must be considered too. Therefore, a vitamin D supplement seems like a better choice.

Q: *I've noticed that many of the calcium supplements sold at my local health food store contain boron—is that good or is it something to avoid?*

A: Some supplements contain a number of trace minerals, including boron. While boron is necessary for bone development, we normally get enough from food. Currently, there is no evidence that boron supplements actually help bone.

Q: *Does the fluoride in my town water supply affect my bones?*

A: We know that fluoride stimulates the osteoblasts, but we're not yet sure how to translate this effect into stronger bones. A few areas of the United States with naturally high levels of fluoride in the water have elevated incidences of hip fractures. (The lower levels of fluoride used in municipal water supplies don't produce this effect.) New fluoride-based bone medications are currently under investigation.

Q: *I have a good diet, but I take a multivitamin supplement just in case. Is there anything wrong with doing that?*

A: No. A multivitamin that supplies 50 to 100 percent of the recommended amounts of vitamins and minerals is safe and could be beneficial. However, I don't recommend that you take a supplement that supplies more than twice the recommended amounts. That's because high levels of one nutrient may interfere with the absorption or metabolism of another.

Does my child get enough calcium?

The DRI for calcium for youngsters ages 4 to 8 is 800 milligrams a day, and 1300 milligrams a day for preadolescents and teens. That's a lot of calcium! Babies and toddlers generally get plenty from milk. But after age 3, most kids don't—and that's a concern because childhood calcium intake is closely related to peak bone mass. Here are some tips to help your child get enough:

- Serve cereal with milk for breakfast.
- Serve milk as a beverage with lunch and dinner.
- Use milk and other dairy foods for snacks—yogurt, pudding, cheese.
- Make high-calcium treats, like fruit smoothies.
- Use calcium-fortified juice and breakfast cereal.

Involve your child in the challenge. Ask her to figure out how to get four servings of calcium-rich foods per day. Maybe she'd like to post a progress chart on the fridge.

Q: *I'm worried about taking vitamin D because I've heard it can be toxic. How can I be sure that I don't get too much?*

A: The established safe upper limit for vitamin D is 2000 international units (IU) per day. It's nearly impossible to get too much from food. But be careful if you're taking multiple supplements—for instance, if you're taking a multivitamin and also a calcium supplement that contains the vitamin. Check the labels and add up the amounts of vitamin D. The total should not be more than 1500 IU per day, since you probably get some vitamin D from food. Unless your doctor has suggested a higher amount, I recommend that you take no more than 600 IU daily.

Q: *I'm 65 years old and I live in Florida. Don't I get enough sun down here so I don't have to take vitamin D?*

A: If you live in Florida, it is possible to produce vitamin D in the skin during the winter months, but the levels are usually lower than in the summer. Also, as we age we synthesize vitamin D much less effectively. So I would still recommend vitamin D supplements for you during the winter months.

I like fruits and vegetables, but I find it hard to get enough because I don't have much time to cook. Any ideas?

It's a common problem. Most of us enjoy eating fruits and vegetables a lot more than we enjoy preparing them. Here are seven ways to make it easy:

- Use ready-to-serve lettuce and veggies to streamline salad preparation.
- Buy cut-up vegetables, such as baby carrots or broccoli flowerets, for convenient snacks.
- Consider the salad bar your assistant chef. Buy vegetables that are already washed and diced or sliced, and add them to stir-fries, soups, stews, and cooked side dishes.
- Drink fruit and vegetable juice; one-portion cans make great snacks for the car or office.
- Keep dried fruit on hand for snacks.
- Top breakfast pancakes or waffles with fruit canned in its own juice.
- Swirl frozen fruit into frozen yogurt or ice cream for snacks or dessert.

Q: *I'm a working mom, and weekday mornings are terribly rushed. Is it okay for me to have a breakfast bar?*

A: Breakfast bars are certainly better than skipping breakfast altogether, so they're fine for occasional emergencies. But if they're becoming a habit, I suggest you make the effort to come up with quick and easy alternatives. Breakfast bars simply don't contain all the nutrients you can get from real food. Grab a piece of fruit and a container of yogurt; slap together a cheese and apple sandwich on whole-grain bread. Or try to rearrange your schedule so you have an extra ten minutes for breakfast.

Q: *Can a high-protein diet harm my bones?*

A: Excess protein consumption—amounts three or four times higher than recommended—can cause loss of bone. This can happen to women who attempt to lose weight by greatly increasing their protein intake. Going to the other extreme isn't good either, because protein is important for bone health. About 30 percent of women don't get enough protein, which adds to their risk for osteoporosis.

EXERCISE

Q: *Which is better—free weights or exercise machines?*

A: Both have their advantages. Exercise machines reduce some potential problems with form and they allow you to lift heavier loads. Free weights, on the other hand, help improve your coordination because they require you to be very aware of your position and body alignment as you do the moves. In addition, free weights are more practical for home use, because they're much smaller and less expensive. I suggest you use whichever you prefer (or have more convenient access to). I myself use both machines and free weights.

Q: *Can I manage with just one ankle weight?*

A: Though it's more convenient to do the leg exercises with two ankle weights, many women follow the program successfully with just one. Instead of alternating legs as they do the leg exercises, they do two sets of each exercise on one leg, then move the weight to the other leg and do another two sets.

Here are two suggestions if you're working with a single ankle weight and doing leg exercises from *Strong Women Stay Young*, which are performed standing:

- Make sure you don't lock the knee of your supporting leg, since that increases stress on the joint.
- If you experience knee pain in the supporting leg, consider investing in another ankle weight.

Q: *My income is limited and I live frugally. Can I make my own weights from detergent bottles or buckets?*

A: For safety's sake, I urge you not to improvise equipment. Detergent bottles and buckets are not designed for strength training and could be unsafe. Two suggestions for economizing: First, check out the sets of dumbbells sold by many sporting goods stores. Often you can save by buying a set and filling in the other weights you need. Another way to economize is to share weights with friends, or to buy used dumbbells.

Q: *Can I use exercise bands instead of heavy weights?*

A: Exercise elastic bands are light and inexpensive. Though bands can be beneficial, it's difficult to follow a progressive program with them (unless you receive proper instruction) and they can be cumbersome to use correctly. Therefore, I prefer dumbbells.

Q: *How long should I wait after eating before exercising?*

A: Ideally, you should wait one to four hours after a meal before working out. Directly following a meal, blood flow is directed toward the stomach for digestion. But when you exercise, blood flows to the muscles. So if you exercise right after you eat, your muscles and your stomach may be shortchanged, which could cause cramping. However, you shouldn't try to exercise on an empty stomach either, because that could leave you feeling drained of energy and fatigued.

Q: *I've read about research that finds one set of twelve reps is enough. Will my bones get the same benefit if I do one set of twelve reps instead of two sets of eight reps?*

A: We're all pressed for time, so it's tempting to cut back on workouts. But before you drop the second set, you need to know some important limitations of these research findings. They're based on programs that differ from the one in this book in two important respects:

First, each workout involved ten or more different exercises. That meant each major muscle group was worked by at least two exercises. So even though the volunteers did just one set per exercise, their muscles received plenty of stimulation.

Second, these programs used strength-training machines, not free weights (dumbbells and ankle weights). Machines hold your body in the correct position. This usually allows you to lift heavier weights.

If you've been doing more than ten different strength-training exercises, you could cut back to one set of eight exercises if time is a problem. However, if you're doing just six to ten exercises, I still recommend that you complete two sets of eight repetitions to get the full benefit for your muscles and bones.

Q: *The instructor at the gym tells me to lift the weight in two seconds and then lower it in four seconds. Is it bad to do it that way?*

A: No, it's fine—provided you lift the weights in a controlled manner. If you swing the weights, your muscles won't get the full benefit of the exercise.

Q: *My left side is weaker than my right. Should I use different weights or wait until my left side catches up?*

A: It's better for both sides of your body to be equal in strength. You can use different weights temporarily, but help your weaker arm to catch up. Advance more slowly—perhaps only every two or three weeks—with your stronger arm, but try to move ahead more quickly with your weaker arm.

Q: *Five pounds isn't challenging enough, but 8 pounds is too much. What should I do?*

A: Make the transition by doing the first set with your 5-pound weights and the second set with the 8-pounders. After a few sessions you should be able to do both sets with the heavier weights.

Q: *Can I do Pilates or yoga instead of strength training?*

A: Yoga and Pilates are terrific exercises that reduce stress and increase both flexibility and coordination, improving your health and fitness. But not all forms of yoga and Pilates provide a strengthening benefit. You can tell by how your muscles feel. If the pose is challenging enough so that you can hold it for only a minute before you need to rest, and if you feel the burn of muscle fatigue, then probably you're getting some strengthening effect. However, it's not likely to be as great as with the strength-training exercises in this book, which work your muscles to fatigue after eight repetitions. If you have osteoporosis, remember that forward flexion can be dangerous to your spine.

Q: *I'm very busy and would like to make my workouts more efficient. Can I lift the weights as I walk?*

A: I sympathize because I'm pressed for time too—but this is not safe. The strength-training program in this book uses weights heavy enough so you can lift them only eight times in good form before you need to rest. The moves require a lot of effort, as well as correct posture (impossible if you're walking) and form. If you're walking, you simply can't give the lifts the kind of concentration they need. There's a real risk that you might injure yourself—if not with the weights, then by tripping as you walk.

Q: I've been making excellent progress—so good that my 20-pound ankle weights are no longer a challenge. Where can I find heavier ones?

A: You can't! Using ankle weights heavier than 20 pounds could create an orthopedic problem. To increase the challenge, switch to more difficult exercises that use your body weight for resistance. (See the list of sources below.) Or work out on strength training machines, which allow you to lift heavier weights safely.

Similarly, don't attempt to lift dumbbells that are heavier than 25 pounds. You can do the biceps curl, overhead press, and upward row with barbells, which are more stable. And again, you can switch to machines.

For more strengthening exercises

See my other books, *Strong Women Stay Young* and *Strong Women Stay Slim*.
Also recommended:
A Woman's Book of Strength, by Karen Andes (Perigee, 1995)
Strength Training for Women, by James A. Peterson, Ph.D. (Human Kinetics, 1995)
Strength Training Past 50, by Wayne Wescott, Ph.D. (Human Kinetics, 1997)

Q: I take an aerobics class that includes twenty minutes of toning—does that count as strength training?

A: No, it doesn't. You're probably getting excellent cardiovascular benefits from the class, but it won't increase your strength. The strengthening workouts in this book involve weights that you can lift only about eight times in good form. If you can easily lift a weight many more times than that, it's not heavy enough to make you stronger or to make a difference for your bones.

I have a special medical concern.

Appropriate exercise can benefit nearly everyone. The research subjects for our exercise studies at Tufts have included frail women with severe osteoporosis, nursing home residents, people who've recovered from major surgery (including joint replacement, hysterectomy, mastectomy, and other cancer treatment), as well as individuals with conditions such as heart disease, diabetes, arthritis, and other joint problems.

The key to success is finding suitable activities. For example, if you have osteoporosis, vertical jumping is not for you. And it's wise to avoid sports that put you at risk for falling. Here are other general recommendations if you have osteoporosis or any other medical condition:

- It's essential to discuss exercise with your doctor before you begin, so you can make any necessary adjustments.
- Start conservatively and progress slowly. For instance, your doctor might suggest that you begin with five minutes of aerobic exercise instead of fifteen, or that you complete your first strengthening workouts without weights. Advancing every other week might be better than trying to add challenge every week.
- Consider scheduling a few sessions with a personal trainer to make sure your form is correct. A trainer can also help you find exercises to meet particular needs.
- Pay attention to your body. If you feel good and have more energy, that's the best indication you're exercising properly.

MEDICATION

Q: *I am 42 years old and I just had a bone density test. The results showed osteoporosis. Now my doctor wants me on Fosamax. I hate to take medication. Can't I do just as well by eating well and getting plenty of exercise?*

A: Because you are young, with many active years ahead of you, I strongly recommend that you take Fosamax, along with eating well and exercising. This combination is the best way to reduce your risk of future fractures.

If you're still not sure about medication, I suggest you try a vigorous exercise program for the coming year, along with a good diet plus calcium and vitamin D supplements. When the year is up, have a bone density test and see where things stand. If you have not seen a benefit—or if you have lost any more bone—I very strongly encourage you to take medication.

Q: *I have breast implants and I am wondering if I can do strength training.*

A: Yes, you can. Talk to your doctor first to make sure there are no special issues that would require you to modify your program. Usually, breast implants are placed above the chest muscles, so strength training should not affect them. But just to be on the safe side, start with low weights and work up very slowly. And don't drop the weights on your chest!

Q: *I recently entered menopause, and my doctor prescribed HRT with a synthetic estrogen. My sister-in-law says that it's better to use a natural estrogen. Does it really make any difference?*

A: Scientific research has not found any difference in effectiveness between natural and synthetic estrogen.

Q: *I'm taking soy isoflavones. Does this mean that I won't need HRT when I reach menopause?*

A: Isoflavones may have a mild beneficial effect on hot flashes and other symptoms of menopause, but they have not been proven to reduce risk of heart disease, osteoporosis, or Alzheimer's—all major reasons why a women might choose HRT. So the decision to go on HRT is not affected by use of isoflavones or other soy products.

Q: *My daughter, who is only 28 years old, was diagnosed with osteoporosis. I know she was hoping to start a family next year. Is there any medication she can take for her bones while she's pregnant?*

A: Unfortunately, no osteoporosis medications have been tested for safety in pregnant women. Since young women may become pregnant unexpectedly, doctors usually don't prescribe Fosamax for them—that's because the drug stays in the body for a long time, and could affect a developing fetus. Your daughter's doctor might suggest nasal calcitonin, which leaves the body very quickly; the doctor is likely to recommend that she go off the medication prior to conception and resume after she stops nursing.

Q: *There's osteoporosis in my family, and I'd like to take HRT, but when I tried it, I got terrible headaches.*

A: Headaches are a common side effect of HRT—but they usually subside after six to nine months. If you can't tolerate the wait, talk to your doctor about trying another prescription or a lower dose of HRT. We're learning that lower doses of estrogen have a positive effect on bone, while reducing side effects. HRT is not recommended for women with a history of migraine headaches since it can exacerbate the problem.

Q: *Will the medication I take for my bones affect the density of my jawbone?*

A: We know that women who take hormone replacement therapy retain more teeth as they age than women who do not go on HRT or estrogen. So you can assume that your medication is helping with bone density in your jaw.

Q: *My bone density is normal in my spine, but I have osteopenia in my hip-bone. I want to know if I should do specific strengthening exercises to help my hip—or does strength training help my entire skeleton?*

A: Exercise helps your hipbones in several different ways. First, the impact of weight-bearing exercise directly stimulates the bones. Second, as the muscles near your hipbones get stronger, they will exert more force upon the bones, providing additional stimulation. And finally, exercise has systemic effects that benefit all the muscles and bones in your body via positive changes in growth factors.

Remember that osteoporosis can affect any bone in the body. That's why the best strengthening exercise program for osteoporosis is a workout that targets the major muscles in the trunk, arms, and legs.

Glossary

Absorptiometry: a technique for measuring bone density by exposing the bone to small amounts of radiation and determining how much is absorbed. Used for dual energy X-ray absorptiometry and single energy X-ray absorptiometry.

Aerobic exercise: physical activity that elevates the heart rate and breathing rate, thereby stimulating the cardiovascular system.

Agonists: drugs with action similar to that of a natural hormone or compound. For example, an estrogen agonist produces effects similar to those of estrogen.

Alendronate: a bisphosphonate (brand name Fosamax) that decreases bone breakdown, which is approved by the FDA for preventing and treating osteoporosis in postmenopausal women.

Amenorrhea: prolonged (usually at least twelve months) absence of a menstrual period in a premenopausal woman who is not pregnant. Causes of amenorrhea include eating disorders, excessive exercise, and medical conditions such as thyroid problems.

Androgens: male hormones, such as testosterone, that are responsible for male sexual characteristics. Women also produce small amounts of androgens.

Anorexia nervosa: a potentially life-threatening psychological disorder in which an individual eats so little that body weight drops to below a BMI of 18 and the menstrual cycle ceases. Most anorectics are young women, but men and older women can be affected too. Intensive psychological help is usually required for successful treatment.

Antacids: medications that decrease the acid in the stomach.

Antiresorptive drugs: medications that decrease activity of the osteoclasts, thereby decreasing bone breakdown.

Biconcave fracture: a spinal fracture in which the upper and lower central portion of the vertebras collapse, but the back and front of the vertebras remain intact.

Bisphosphonates: a type of medication that decreases the activity of osteoclasts, thereby decreasing bone breakdown. Alendronate (Fosamax) is a bisphosphonate.

Body mass index (BMI): the ratio of weight in kilograms to height in meters, which is used to assess body weight. BMI between 19 and 25 is considered healthy.

Bone densitometry: measurement of bone density. (See *absorptiometry*.)

Bone density or bone-mineral density (BMD): the amount of mineralized bone tissue in a given area of bone, usually expressed as grams per centimeter squared (g/cm^2) or, in the case of three-dimensional CT scans, milligrams per centimeter cubed (mg/cm^3).

Bone mass: the total amount of bone mineral in the body.

Bone remodeling: the cycle of bone growth, maintenance, and repair, in which the osteoclasts dissolve old bone and new bone tissue is built by the osteoblasts.

Calcitonin: a naturally occurring hormone that inhibits osteoclast (bone breakdown) activity. Calcitonin is available in drug form (brand name Miacalcin) and is approved by the FDA for treatment of osteoporosis.

Calcitriol: a synthetic form of vitamin D, which can be toxic. It does not have FDA approval for treatment or prevention of osteoporosis.

Calcium: a mineral found in dairy products and other foods that plays an essential role in bone development and health, as well as in other vital functions of the body.

Calcium carbonate: one of several calcium compounds used in nutritional supplements.

Calcium citrate: one of several calcium compounds used in nutritional supplements.

Collagen: a protein that is the chief component of cartilage, skin, and connective tissue, as well as an important part of bone.

Colles' fracture: a common type of wrist fracture, in which the radial bone is broken.

Compression fracture: a fracture of the spine in which the entire vertebra collapses. Also, known as a crush fracture.

Computerized axial tomography (CT or CAT): a three-dimensional X ray that can measure bone density.

Conjugated equine estrogen: a mixture of estrogens formulated from the urine of pregnant mares (brand name Premarin), one of the forms of estrogen replacement therapy approved by the FDA for prevention and treatment of osteoporosis.

Control group: a group of research volunteers who do not receive the intervention being tested, so the effects of the intervention can be assessed.

Cortical bone: the dense outer layer of bone tissue.

Corticosteroids: hormones produced by the adrenal glands, or drugs such as cortisone that resemble adrenal hormones. These drugs—which are used to treat asthma, arthritis, and other diseases—can have adverse effects on bone.

Cortisone: a hormone produced by the adrenal glands that can be detrimental to bone. (See *corticosteroids.*)

Cytokines: hormonelike compounds that help regulate immune response and that also play a role in the regulation of osteoblasts and osteoclasts.

Daidzein: a type of isoflavone found in soybeans that is thought to be beneficial to bone.

Daily Value (DV): nutrition guidelines developed by the FDA specifically for use on food labels.

Dietary Reference Intake (DRI): guidelines from the Food and Nutrition Board of the National Academy of Sciences for the daily nutrient intake for a healthy diet.

Diuretics: drugs that promote urine excretion.

Dowager's hump: see *kyphosis.*

Dual energy X-ray absorptiometry (DXA or DEXA): the method most commonly used to measure bone density. DXA can precisely measure total bone density in the body, as well as the density of bones in the hip, spine, and arm.

Elemental calcium: the actual amount of calcium contained in a compound, such as a nutritional supplement. About 40 percent of calcium carbonate, and 21 percent of calcium citrate, is elemental calcium.

Endometriosis: a sometimes painful condition in which endometrial tissue—tissue from the lining of the uterus—grows elsewhere in the abdomen, such as on the surface of the uterus, fallopian tubes, or ovaries.

Estradiol: the most potent form of naturally occurring estrogen.

Estrogen: female sex hormones, including estradiol, estrone, and estriol.

Estrogen replacement therapy (ERT): treatment in which estrogen is given to postmenopausal women. See also *hormone replacement therapy (HRT),* in which progesterone is given along with estrogen. ERT usually is recommended only for women whose uterus has been removed, because treatment with estrogen alone is linked to increased rates of endometrial cancer.

Etidronate: a type of bisphosphonate that decreases the rate of bone remodeling. Etidronate has FDA approval for treatment of Paget's disease, a rare bone disorder, but does not yet have FDA approval for prevention or treatment of osteoporosis.

Evista: see *raloxifene.*

Femur: the long bone of the thigh—the longest bone in the body.

Fluoride: a naturally occurring element that stimulates formation of bone and teeth. Fluoride is added to the water supply in many communities to reduce tooth decay. Studies are under way to assess the value of fluoride in different forms for treating and preventing osteoporosis.

Follicle-stimulating hormone (FSH): hormone produced in the pituitary gland that helps regulate the menstrual cycle. Blood FSH levels, which usually rise as women go through menopause, are used to check menopausal status.

Food and Drug Administration (FDA): an agency within the United States Department of Health and Human Services' Public Health Service that is responsible for ensuring the safety and efficacy of medications, as well as all foods (except meat, poultry, and eggs), that are processed and sold in interstate commerce. Meat, poultry, and eggs are regulated by the United States Department of Agriculture.

Fosamax: see *alendronate.*

Genistein: an isoflavone that occurs naturally in soybeans and is thought to be beneficial to bone.

Growth factors: compounds in the body, including growth hormone, that are responsible for the growth, repair, and regeneration of various tissues, including bone.

Growth hormone: a hormone produced by the pituitary gland that stimulates the growth of many tissues in the body, including bone.

Hip fracture: any fracture of the femur bone in or around the hip joint.

Hormone replacement therapy (HRT): treatment for postmenopausal women in which estrogen is given along with progesterone, either cyclically or continuously. HRT is generally prescribed for women who still have a uterus, and who would be at elevated risk for endometrial cancer if they used estrogen alone.

Hormones: chemicals produced by cells and transported via the bloodstream to other cells and organs in the body, on which they have specific effects.

Hot flash or hot flush: a sensation of sudden warmth, often accompanied by sweating, that is caused by dilation of blood vessels. This is a common symptom of menopause.

Hysterectomy: surgical removal of the uterus and cervix. The term "complete hysterectomy" is used when the ovaries are removed as well.

Impact-loading exercise: a physical activity, such as jumping rope or vertical jumping, that produces a significant amount of force on bone.

Ipriflavone: a synthetic compound derived from natural isoflavones that has been shown to be beneficial to bone.

Isoflavone: a natural plant compound found mainly in soy foods that produces estrogenlike effects in the body.

Kyphosis: outward curvature of the upper part of the spine, caused by collapsed vertebras, that produces stooped-over posture as well as protuberance of the upper back. Sometimes called "dowager's hump."

Lactose intolerance: inability to digest lactose, the naturally occurring sugar in dairy products, because an individual has insufficient amounts of the enzyme lactase. Symptoms include gastrointestinal discomfort, gas, and diarrhea after eating dairy products that contain lactose.

Lumbar spine: the five vertebras that comprise the lower part of the spine.

Magnesium: an essential mineral, contained in food, used for different biochemical processes in the body, including bone formation.

Mammogram: a diagnostic X-ray procedure used to detect breast cancer.

Menarche: the onset of menstruation at puberty. Girls normally reach menarche between age 11 and 16.

Menopause: cessation of menstruation, usually occurring between age 45 and 55 as the ovaries produce less estrogen and progesterone.

Miacalcin: see *calcitonin.*

Osteoblasts: cells responsible for bone formation.

Osteoclasts: cells responsible for bone breakdown.

Osteopenia: bone density that is abnormally low, but not low enough to be classified as osteoporosis. Now defined as bone density between 1 and 2.5 standard deviations below the mean for young normal adults (T-score between −1 and −2.5).

Osteoporosis: a chronic, progressive disease characterized by low bone mass, leading to bone fragility and increased fracture risk. For diagnostic purposes, a bone density more than 2.5 standard deviations below the mean for normal young adults (T-score below −2.5).

Ovary: the almond-shaped organ in women that produces estrogen and eggs.

Ovulation: release of the mature egg by the ovary. This usually occurs in the middle of the menstrual cycle.

Oxalates: compounds present in foods, especially green vegetables, that can bind calcium (and other minerals), thereby interfering with their absorption in the body.

Parathyroid hormone (PTH): a hormone released by the parathyroid glands in response to low blood levels of calcium, which stimulates breakdown of bone. In drug form PTH is sometimes used to treat osteoporosis, although it does not yet have FDA approval for this purpose.

Peak bone mass: the highest amount of bone mass a person has during his or her lifetime. Peak bone mass is usually achieved in young adulthood.

Phosphorus: an essential mineral, found in food, which is essential for many chemical processes in the body and is also a component of bones and teeth.

Phytoestrogens: compounds found in plants that have estrogenlike effects in the body.

Pituitary gland: a small gland at the base of the brain that produces FSH, thyroid-stimulating hormone, and other key hormones of the body.

Placebo: an inert, harmless substance, such as sugar pills, given to the control group in research studies. Effects of the actual treatment are compared to the effects of the placebo.

Premarin: see *conjugated equine estrogen.*

Progesterone: a female hormone produced by the ovaries in the second half of the menstrual cycle and during pregnancy. In hormone replacement therapy, progesterone is added to estrogen to reduce the risk of endometrial cancer.

Proprioception: the ability to know where one is in space.

Prostaglandins: biologically active compounds that are synthesized in the body from fatty acids, which affect bone formation, blood pressure, action of smooth muscles, fluid balance, blood flow, body temperature, blood clotting, and other functions.

Quadriceps: four muscles in the front of each thigh, which govern forward movement and straightening of the lower leg.

Radius: the bone of the forearm that extends from the base of the thumb to the elbow.

Raloxifene: a selective estrogen receptor modulator (SERM), or weak estrogen. Has FDA approval for preventing and treating osteoporosis, and also is believed to reduce the risk of breast cancer.

Randomization: in research studies, an unbiased process for selecting members of the treatment and control groups.

Receptor: the area on the surface of a cell that responds to a substance. Most hormones have a specific receptor that must be present on the cell in order for the hormone to exert its effects.

Remodeling: see *bone remodeling*.

Resistance exercise: a mode of physical activity in which the muscle works against a force provided by free weights, machines, or body weight.

Resorption: the breakdown phase of the bone remodeling process, in which bone is lost.

Selective estrogen receptor modulators (SERMs): compounds that have estrogenlike effects on the body, often without the negative side effects of estrogen. Some SERMs, including tamoxifen and raloxifene, have positive effects on bone.

Steroids: anti-inflammatory medications used to treat medical problems such as asthma, arthritis, and chronic dermatitis. Can have a negative effect on bone.

Strength training: a mode of resistance exercise in which the muscle works against a resistance sufficiently high to increase strength.

Surgical menopause: cessation of menstruation caused by removal of the ovaries prior to natural menopause.

T-score: a statistical measure indicating the difference between an individual's score and the mean score of a relevant population. With bone density, used to compare scores to the bone-mineral density of normal young adults, and to classify people as having normal bone density, osteopenia, or osteoporosis.

Tamoxifen: a SERM used to treat breast cancer, which has some positive effects on bone but is not used to treat or prevent osteoporosis.

Target heart rate: heart rate recommended as a target for individuals doing aerobic exercise.

Testosterone: see *androgens*.

Thiazides: a type of diuretic used to treat high blood pressure, which conserves calcium in the kidney. Believed to be beneficial to bone, but not used for treating or preventing osteoporosis.

Thoracic spine: the twelve vertebras that comprise the middle part of the spine.

Thyroid: the organ in the neck that produces thyroid hormones, which control metabolism. High levels of thyroid hormones are detrimental to bone.

Trabecular bone: lacy structure of calcium crystals inside bone, under the hard layer of cortical bone.

Trace minerals: essential minerals—such as iron, zinc, and selenium—that are found in the human body in tiny amounts (less than 5 grams).

Trochanter: the top outside of the femur bone.

Ultrasound: high-frequency sound waves, which can create images of bone and other structures within the body. Used to assess bone density at the heel or knee.

Vertebras: the cylindrical bones that make up the spine, which are frequent sites of osteoporotic fractures.

Vitamins: nutrients found in plant and animal foods that are required by the body in small amounts for normal growth and function.

Ward's triangle: area in the central part of the upper hipbone (femur) that is usually measured during DXA tests of hipbone density.

Wedge fracture: a vertebral fracture in which only the front of the vertebra fractures; the back of the vertebra remains intact. This type of fracture contributes to kyphosis.

Weight-bearing exercise: a mode of physical activity, such as walking, in which the legs support the weight of the body.

Weight training: see *resistance exercise.*

Z-score: a statistical measure indicating the difference between an individual's score and the mean score of a relevant population. With bone density, Z-scores are used to compare individuals to the mean of normal adults of the same age.

References

◆ ◆ ◆

Below is a partial list of the scientific articles I used as I researched the medical literature for this book. If you are interested in reading any of them, I suggest you contact the reference librarian at your local public library for assistance. Some of the journals are available from large public or university libraries; others can be read at medical school libraries.

Osteoporosis

Albright, F., P. Smith and A. Richardson (1941). "Postmenopausal osteoporosis." *Journal of the American Medical Association* 116(22): 2465–2474.

Cook, D., G. Guyatt, J. Adachi, J. Clifton, L. Griffith, R. Epstein and E. Juniper (1993). "Quality of life issues in women with vertebral fractures due to osteoporosis." *Arthritis and Rheumatism* 36(6): 750–756.

Eddy, D., C. Johnston, S. Cummings, B. Dawson-Hughes, R. Lindsay, L. Melton and C. Slemenda (1998). "Osteoporosis: review of the evidence for prevention, diagnosis and treatment and cost-effectiveness analysis." *Osteoporosis International* 8(S4): 1–88.

Kanis, J., J. Melton, C. Christiansen, C. Johnston and N. Khaltaev (1994). "The diagnosis of osteoporosis." *Journal of Bone and Mineral Research* 9(8): 1137–1141.

Kannus, P., J. Parkkari, H. Sievanen, A. Heinonen, I. Vuori and M. Jarvinen (1996). "Epidemiology of hip fractures." *Bone* 18(1S): 57S–63S.

Melton, L. (1996). "Epidemiology of hip fractures: implications of the exponential increase with age." *Bone* 18(3S): 121S–125S.

Wasnich, R. (1996). "Vertebral fracture epidemiology." *Bone* 18(3S): 179S–183S.

Risk factors

Cummings, S., M. Nevitt, W. Browner, K. Stone, K. Fox, K. Ensrud, J. Cauley, D. Black and T. Vogt (1995). "Risk factors for hip fractures in white women." *New England Journal of Medicine* 332(12): 767–773.

Harris, S. (1997). "Effects of caffeine consumption on hip fracture, bone density and calcium retention." *Nutritional Aspects of Osteoporosis.* In P. Burckhardt, B. Dawson-Hughes and R. Heaney. New York, Springer-Verlag: 163–171.

Krall, E. and B. Dawson-Hughes (1991). "Smoking and bone loss among post-menopausal women." *Journal of Bone and Mineral Research* 6(4): 331–337.

Michaelsson, K., J. Baron, B. Farahmand, I. Persson and S. Ljunghall (1999). "Oral-contraceptive use and risk of hip fracture: a case-control study." *Lancet* 353: 1481–1484.

Falls

Buchner, D., M. Cress, B. de Lateur, P. Esselman, A. Margherita, R. Price and E. Wagner (1997). "The effect of strength and endurance training on gait, balance, fall risk, and health services use in community-living older adults." *Journal of Gerontology* 52A(4): M218–M224.

Campbell, A., M. Borrie and G. Spears (1989). "Risk factors for falls in a community-based prospective study of people 70 years and older." *Journal of Gerontology* 44(4): M112–117.

Campbell, A., M. Robertson, M. Gardner, R. Norton, M. Tilyard and D. Buchner (1997). "Randomized controlled trial of a general practice programme of home-based exercise to prevent falls in elderly women." *British Medical Journal* 315: 1065–1069.

Hindmarsh, J. and H. Estes (1989). "Falls in older persons: causes and interventions." *Archives of Internal Medicine* 149: 2217–2222.

Tinetti, M., D. Baker, G. McAvay, E. Claus, P. Garrett, M. Gottschalk, M. Koch, K. Trainor and R. Horwitz (1994). "A multifactorial intervention to reduce the risk of falling among elderly people living in the community." *New England Journal of Medicine* 331(13): 822–827.

Nutrition

Bingham, S., C. Atkinson, J. Liggins, L. Bluck and A. Coward (1998). "Phyto-estrogens: where are we now?" *British Journal of Nutrition* 79(5): 393–406.

Buckley, L., E. Leib, K. Cartularo, P. Vacek and S. Cooper (1996). "Calcium and vitamin D_3 supplementation prevents bone loss in the spine secondary to low-dose corticosteroids in patients with rheumatoid arthritis: a randomized, double-blind, placebo-controlled trial." *Annals of Internal Medicine* 125: 961–968.

Dawson-Hughes, B. (1991). "Calcium supplementation and bone loss: a review of controlled clinical trials." *American Journal of Clinical Nutrition* 54: 274S–280S.

Dawson-Hughes, B., G. Dallal, E. Krall, S. Harris, L. Sokoll and G. Falconer (1991). "Effect of vitamin D supplementation on wintertime and overall bone loss in healthy postmenopausal women." *Annals of Internal Medicine* 115: 505–512.

Dawson-Hughes, B., G. Dallal, E. Krall, L. Sadowski, N. Sahyoun and S. Tannenbaum (1990). "A controlled trial of the effect of calcium supplementation on bone density in postmenopausal women." *New England Journal of Medicine* 323(13): 878–883.

Dawson-Hughes, B. and S. Harris (1992). "Regional changes in body composition by time of year in healthy postmenopausal women." *American Journal of Clinical Nutrition* 56: 307–313.

Dawson-Hughes, B., S. Harris, E. Krall and G. Dallal (1997). "Effect of calcium and vitamin D supplementation on bone density in men and women 65 years of age or older." *New England Journal of Medicine* 337: 670–676.

Feskanich, D., P. Weber, W. Willett, H. Rockett, S. Booth and G. Colditz (1999). "Vitamin K intake and hip fractures in women: a prospective study." *American Journal of Clinical Nutrition* 69: 74–79.

Matkovic, V., K. Kostial, I. Simonovic, R. Buzina, A. Brodarec and B. Nordin (1979). "Bone status and fracture rates in two regions of Yugoslavia." *American Journal of Clinical Nutrition* 32: 540–549.

Potter, S., J. Baum, H. Teng, R. Stillman, N. Shay and J. Erdman (1998). "Soy protein and isoflavones: their effects on blood lipids and bone density in postmenopausal women." *American Journal of Clinical Nutrition* 68 (Supplement): 1375S–1379S.

Teegarden, D., R. Lyle, W. Proulx, C. Johnston and C. Weaver (1999). "Previous milk consumption is associated with greater bone density in young women." *American Journal of Clinical Nutrition* 69: 1014–1017.

Tilyard, M., G. Spears, J. Thomson and S. Dovey (1992). "Treatment of postmenopausal osteoporosis with calcitriol or calcium." *New England Journal of Medicine* 326(6): 357–362.

Tucker, K., M. Hannan, H. Chen, L. Cupples, P. Wilson and D. Kiel (1999). "Potassium, magnesium, and fruit and vegetable intakes are associated with greater bone mineral density in elderly men and women." *American Journal of Clinical Nutrition* 69: 727–736.

Exercise

Bassey, E. and S. Ramsdale (1994). "Increase in femoral bone density in young women following high-impact exercise." *Osteoporosis International* 4(2): 72–75.

Drinkwater, B., K. Nilson, C. Chesnut, W. Bremner, S. Shainholtz and M. Southworth (1984). "Bone mineral content of amenorrheic and eumenorrheic athletes." *New England Journal of Medicine* 311(5): 277–281.

Fehling, P., L. Alekel, J. Clasey, A. Rector and R. Stillman (1995). "A comparison of bone mineral densities among female athletes in impact loading and active loading sports." *Bone* 17(3): 205–210.

Fisher, E., M. Nelson, W. Frontera, R. Turksoy and W. Evans (1986). "Bone mineral content and levels of gonadotropins and estrogens in amenorrheic running women." *Journal of Clinical Endocrinology and Metabolism* 62: 1232–1236.

Kohrt, W., A. Ehsani and S. Birge (1997). "Effects of exercise involving predominantly either joint-reaction or ground-reaction forces on bone mineral density in older women." *Journal of Bone and Mineral Research* 12(8): 1253–1261.

Kohrt, W., A. Ehsani and S. Birge (1998). "HRT preserves increases in bone mineral density and reductions in body fat after a supervised exercise program." *Journal of Applied Physiology* 84(5): 1506–1512.

Layne, J. and M. Nelson (1999). "The effects of progressive resistance training on bone density: a review." *Medicine and Science in Sports and Exercise* 31(1): 25–30.

Morris, F., A. Geraldine, J. Gibbs, J. Carlson and J. Wark (1997). "Prospective tenmonth exercise intervention in premenarcheal girls: positive effects on bone and lean mass." *Journal of Bone and Mineral Research* 12(9): 1453–1462.

Nelson, M., M. Fiatarone, C. Morganti, I. Trice, R. Greenberg and W. Evans (1994). "Effects of high-intensity strength training on multiple risk factors for osteoporotic fractures." *Journal of the American Medical Association* 272: 1900–1914.

Nelson, M., E. Fisher, F. Dilmanian, G. Dallal and W. Evans (1991). "A 1-year walking program and increased dietary calcium in postmenopausal women: effects on bone." *American Journal of Clinical Nutrition* 53: 1394–1411.

Nelson, M., E. Fisher, P. Catsos, C. Meredith, R. Turksoy and W. Evans (1986). "Diet and bone status in amenorrheic runners." *American Journal of Clinical Nutrition* 43: 910–916.

Notelovitz, M., D. Martin, R. Tesar et al. (1991). "Estrogen therapy and variable resistance weight training increases bone mineral in surgically menopausal
women." *Journal of Bone and Mineral Research* 6: 583–590.

Shaw, J. and C. Snow (1998). "Weighted vest exercise improves indices of fall risk
in older women." *Journal of Gerontology* 53(1): M53–M58.

Snow-Harter, C. and M. Bouxsein (1992). "Effects of resistance and endurance exercise on bone mineral status of young women: a randomized exercise intervention trial." *Journal of Bone and Mineral Research* 7(7): 761–769.

Specker, B. (1996). "Evidence for an interaction between calcium intake and physical activity on changes in bone mineral density." *Journal of Bone and Mineral
Research* 11(10): 1539–1544.

Taaffe, D., T. Robinson, C. Snow and R. Marcus (1997). "High-impact exercise promotes bone gain in well-trained female athletes." *Journal of Bone and Mineral
Research* 12(2): 255–260.

Medications

Black, D., S. Cummings, D. Karpf, J. Cauley, D. Thompson, M. Nevitt, D. Bauer, H.
Genant, W. Haskell, R. Marcus, S. Oft, J. Torner, S. Quandt et al. (1996). "Randomized trial of effect of alendronate on risk of fracture in women with existing vertebral fractures." *Lancet* 348: 1535–1541.

Col, N., M. Eckman, R. Karis, S. Pauker, R. Goldberg, E. Ross, R. Orr and J. Wong
(1997). "Patient-specific decisions about hormone replacement therapy in postmenopausal women." *New England Journal of Medicine* 277(14): 1140–1147.

Col, N., S. Pauker, R. Goldberg, M. Eckman, R. Orr, E. Ross and J. Wong (1999).
"Individualizing therapy to prevent long-term consequences of estrogen deficiency in postmenopausal women." *New England Journal of Medicine* 159(13):
1458–1466.

Cummings, S., D. Black, D. Thompson, W. Applegate, E. Barrett-Connor, T.
Musliner, L. Palermo, R. Prineas, S. Rubin, J. Scott, T. Vogt, R. Wallace, J. Yates
et al. (1998). "Effect of alendronate on risk of fracture in women with low bone
density but without vertebral fractures: results from the fracture intervention
trial." *Journal of the American Medical Association* 280(24): 2077–2082.

Cummings, S., S. Eckert, K. Krueger, D. Grady, T. Powles, J. Cauley, L. Norton, T.
Nickelsen, N. Bjarnason, M. Morrow, M. Lippman, D. Black, J. Glusman et al.
(1999). "The effect of raloxifene on risk of breast cancer in postmenopausal
women: results from the MORE randomized trial." *Journal of the American
Medical Association* 281(23): 2189–2197.

Ettinger, B., D. Black, B. Mitlak, R. Knickerbocker, T. Nickelsen, H. Genant, C. Christiansen, P. Delmas, J. Zanchetta, J. Stakkestad, C. Gluer, K. Krueger, F. Cohen et al. (1999). "Reduction of vertebral fracture risk in postmenopausal women with osteoporosis treated with raloxifene." *Journal of the American Medical Association* 282(7): 637–645.

Felson, D., Y. Zhang, M. Hannan, D. Kiel, P. Wilson and J. Anderson (1993). "The effect of postmenopausal estrogen therapy on bone density in elderly women." *New England Journal of Medicine* 329(16): 1141–1146.

Gambacciani, M., M. Ciaponi, L. Cappagli, L. Piaggesi, R. De Simone, R. Orlandi and Genazzani (1997). "Body weight, body fat distribution, and hormonal replacement therapy in early postmenopausal women." *Journal of Clinical Endocrinology and Metabolism* 82(2): 414–417.

Keating, N., P. Cleary, A. Rossi, A. Zaslavsky and J. Ayanian (1999). "Use of hormone replacement by postmenopausal women in the United States." *Annals of Internal Medicine* 130: 545–553.

Recker, R., K. Davies, R. Dowd and R. Heaney (1999). "The effect of low-dose continuous estrogen and progesterone therapy with calcium and vitamin D on bone in elderly women: a randomized, controlled trial." *Annals of Internal Medicine* 130: 897–904.

Reginster, J., L. Meurmans, B. Zegels, L. Rovati, H. Minne, G. Giacovelli, A. Taquet, I. Setnikar, J. Collette and C. Gosset (1998). "The effects of sodium monofluorophosphate plus calcium on vertebral fracture rate in postmenopausal women with moderate osteoporosis: a randomized, controlled trial." *Annals of Internal Medicine* 129(1): 1–8.

Index

About Miriam E. Nelson and Sarah Wernick
authors of *Strong Women Stay Slim* and
Strong Women Stay Young

Miriam E. Nelson, Ph.D., is Associate Professor of Nutrition and Director of the Center for Physical Fitness at the School of Nutrition Science and Policy at Tufts University. She is a Fellow of the American College of Sports Medicine and holds their certification as a Health/Fitness Director. Her original research papers on bone density and physical activity have been published in distinguished peer-reviewed journals, including the *Journal of the American Medical Association*. In 1994 she was named a Brookdale National Fellow; this prestigious award is given annually to only five or six young scholars in the field of aging. She was a Bunting Fellow at Radcliffe College in 1997–1998. Dr. Nelson serves on the Advisory Committee for the Massachusetts Osteoporosis Awareness Program. She lives in Concord, Massachusetts, with her husband and three children.

Sarah Wernick, Ph.D., is an award-winning freelance writer based in Brookline, Massachusetts. Her articles have appeared in *Woman's Day, Working Mother, Smithsonian,* the *New York Times,* and other publications. She is married and has two children.

The *Strong Women* World Wide Web site is
http://www.strongwomen.com.